Student Workbook for

Pharmacology Made Simple
An Introduction for the Health Professions

Anthony Guerra, PharmD

Chemistry Instructor
Pre-Pharmacy Advisor
Former Chair, Pharmacy Technician Program
Des Moines Area Community College
Ankeny, IA

ELSEVIER

ELSEVIER

3251 Riverport Lane
St. Louis, Missouri 63043

STUDENT WORKBOOK FOR PHARMACOLOGY MADE SIMPLE   ISBN: 978-0-323-69576-3

ISBN: 978-0-323-69576-3

Content Strategist: Kristin Wilhelm
Content Development Specialist: Jeannine Carrado
Publishing Services Manager: Deepthi Unni
Project Manager: Haritha Dharmarajan
Design Direction: Patrick Ferguson

Working together
to grow libraries in
developing countries

www.elsevier.com • www.bookaid.org

Printed in the United States of America

Last digit is the print number: 9 8 7 6 5 4 3 2 1

Contents

Chapter 1	Introduction to Pharmacology	1
Chapter 2	Drug Actions (Pharmacodynamics)	5
Chapter 3	Drug Movement (Pharmacokinetics)	11
Chapter 4	Drug Laws and Preventing Medication Errors	17
Chapter 5	Drug Administration	21
Chapter 6	Dosage Calculations	27
Chapter 7	Drug Classifications	31
Chapter 8	Gastrointestinal	35
Chapter 9	Musculoskeletal	41
Chapter 10	Respiratory	47
Chapter 11	Immune	53
Chapter 12	Neuropsychology	61
Chapter 13	Cardiology	69
Chapter 14	Endocrine	77
Chapter 15	PediatricPharmacology	85
Chapter 16	GeriatricPharmacology	91
Chapter 17	Local and General Anesthetics	95
Chapter 18	Alcohol and Drugs of Abuse	103

1 Introduction to Pharmacology

TRUE FALSE (10)

1. Pathophysiology is the study of drugs and their actions. _____
2. An over-the-counter (OTC) drug is safe for most people to take independently, as determined by the FDA. _____
3. Prescription drugs (Rx) do not require a physician to prescribe them. _____
4. Schedule IV medications have a high potential for abuse. _____
5. Currently, there is no accepted medical use for medications in Schedule I. _____
6. Ibuprofen is the brand name, and Advil is the generic name. _____
7. Medications that are not scheduled have a limit of five refills in 6 months. _____
8. Behind-the-counter (BTC) medications are usually found closer to the cash register rather than on the shelf with OT C medicines. _____
9. Generic or nonproprietary drug names are used instead of chemical names because it is too cumbersome. _____
10. Schedules I, II, III, IV, and V that the DEA created are listed from most addictive to least addictive. _____

MULTIPLE CHOICE (10)

1. Which would fall into DEA Schedule I with no accepted medical use and illegal to possess?
   a. heroin
   b. fentanyl (Duragesic)
   c. buprenorphine (Suboxone)
   d. diazepam (Valium)

2. How many months of refills are allowed for a DEA Schedule II prescription for hydrocodone/acetaminophen (Vicodin, Lortab)?
   a. 0
   b. 3
   c. 6
   d. 12

3. A student can best describe pathophysiology as the:
   a. biology of healthy states.
   b. chemistry course before pharmacology.
   c. study of drugs and their actions.
   d. the study of disease in living organisms.

4. Examples of the proper way to write a generic and brand name at the beginning of a sentence would look like which of the following? *(Select all that apply.)*
   a. Ibuprofen (Motrin)
   b. Acetaminophen, Tylenol
   c. Magnesium hydroxide (Milk of Magnesia)
   d. Tums, Calcium carbonate

5. Which OTC medication is *not* recommended for a patient who is prone to ulceration?
   a. omeprazole (Prilosec OTC)
   b. pantoprazole (Prevacid 24HR)
   c. ibuprofen (Advil, Motrin)
   d. acetaminophen (Tylenol)

1

6. The DEA schedule that lists drugs most likely to cause dependence and abuse for which a patient can have no refills is:
   a. Schedule II.
   b. Schedule III.
   c. Schedule IV.
   d. Schedule V.

7. When looking for OTC Advil, we expect that the generic name of the active ingredient will be:
   a. ibuprofen.
   b. pseudoephedrine.
   c. acetaminophen.
   d. phenylephrine.

8. Ciprofloxacin includes which element of the periodic table of elements in its drug name?
   a. hydrogen
   b. chlorine
   c. fluorine
   d. sulfur

9. Which is an OTC medication?
   a. albuterol (ProAir)
   b. methotrexate (Rheumatrex)
   c. calcium carbonate (Tums)
   d. amoxicillin (Amoxil)

10. All are generic names *except*:
   a. calcium carbonate.
   b. (RS)-2-(4-(2-methylpropyl)phenyl) propanoic acid.
   c. ibuprofen.
   d. magnesium hydroxide.

MATCHING (5)

Match the chemical branches to the drug name by looking closely at the generic drug name.

1. _____ acetyl	a. acetaminophen
2. _____ disulfide	b. furosemide
3. _____ furan	c. levetiracetam
4. _____ alcohol	d. tramadol
5. _____ acetyl and phenol	e. disulfiram

COMPLETION (5)

1. Oxycodone (OxyContin) is an example of a _____ medication.

2. Possession of a _____ drug can be illegal.

3. Acetaminophen with codeine (Tylenol #3) and buprenorphine (Suboxone) are _____ medications.

4. On this list, the _____ medicines have the least potential for abuse.

5. Medications that are _____ can include antianxiety or some muscle relaxant medications.

a. Schedule I
b. Schedule II
c. Schedule IV
d. Schedule V
e. Schedule III

DOSAGE CALCULATIONS (5)

1. A patient is prescribed two 200 mg tablets every 6 hours. How many milligrams would the patient take in 24 hours?

2. Acetaminophen has a limit of 2000 mg in a day for patients with liver issues or alcoholism. How many 650-mg acetaminophen extra-strength tablets can they take in a day without exceeding the limit?

3. A patient is prescribed 30 tablets a month and has five refills left. How many total tablets does the prescription call for over 6 months?

4. A provider can convert Duragesic 50 micrograms (mcg) to milligrams (mg). If there are 1000 micrograms in a milligram, how many milligrams is 50 mcg of Duragesic?

5. There are 180 mcg of albuterol in every two puffs. How many mcg of medicine will a patient take if they use two puffs every 6 hours for a single day? How many milligrams will that number represent?

2 Drug Actions (Pharmacodynamics)

TRUE FALSE (10)

1. Systemic effects are when the therapeutic or toxic effect limits itself to a single site. _____
2. The dose required to keep the therapeutic level is the maintenance dose. _____
3. A toxic dose is the one that kills the patient. _____
4. Pharmacodynamics is the study of drug actions or the effect the drug has on the body. _____
5. Drugs will often work to minimize the therapeutic effect and maximize the adverse reactions. _____
6. Agonists are substances that block receptors, which prevents the receptor's activation. _____
7. An allosteric site is when a noncompetitive antagonist binds to it. _____
8. The TD_{50} is the effective dose for 50% of the population taking the drug. _____
9. When a drug has a small margin between the safe and dangerous dose, it has a narrow therapeutic index. _____
10. A high therapeutic index expresses the larger gap between the safe and dangerous dose. _____

MULTIPLE CHOICE (10)

1. What is the effect of a patient using a topical cream to relieve pain in their knee?
   a. local effect
   b. adverse effect
   c. systemic effect
   d. toxic effect

2. The way to express the effectiveness of an individual dose of a drug would be _____.
   a. ED_{25}
   b. TD_{50}
   c. ED_{50}
   d. TD_{25}

3. What types of hormones and medications come from animals and fungi? *(Select all that apply.)*
   a. thyroid
   b. monoclonal antibodies
   c. insulin
   d. antibiotics

4. Based on the therapeutic index, which drug would be the safest to give to a patient?
   a. drug 1 with a therapeutic index of 5
   b. drug 2 with a therapeutic index of 2
   c. drug 3 with a therapeutic index of 8
   d. drug 4 with a therapeutic index of 7

5. If phenytoin (Dilantin), an antiepileptic, has a narrow therapeutic index, which therapeutic index number would indicate this?
   a. 5
   b. 6
   c. 7
   d. 8

6. Which would make this statement correct? A drug with _____ attraction to a receptor would have _____ affinity.
   a. high; low
   b. strong; high
   c. low; high
   d. weak; high

7. What kind of drug provides a weak pharmacologic response?
   a. full agonist
   b. competitive antagonist
   c. partial agonist
   d. noncompetitive antagonist

8. A patient receives a loading dose of two tablets on the first day. What would we call a regimen of one tablet each day for 5 days after the first day?
   a. bolus dose
   b. toxic dose
   c. adverse effect dose
   d. maintenance dose

9. Adverse drug reactions:
   a. limit themselves to a single site.
   b. have an undesired harmful effect.
   c. cause a maximum response.
   d. do not affect the body.

10. What is the therapeutic index when a drug has TD_{50} of 50 and an ED_{50} of 10?
    a. 500
    b. 50
    c. 40
    d. 5

MATCHING (5)

Match the drug activity to the type of drug.

1. _____ The drug binds to the same site as an agonist but does not activate it.

2. _____ The drug will move away and the agonist will act later.

3. _____ The drug binds to an allosteric site to prevent receptor activation.

4. _____ The drug causes a maximal response.

5. _____ The drug binds to the receptor but produces a weak response.

a. full agonist
b. partial agonist
c. competitive antagonist
d. noncompetitive antagonist
e. reversible antagonist

COMPLETION (5)

1. A _____ occurs when patients use topical products to limit toxic effects to a single site.

2. A patient received a _____, which caused significant adverse effects.

3. A patient will usually receive a _____ to raise drug levels quickly, often on the first day.

4. Unfortunately, some patients have died because they ingested a _____.

5. Sometimes, drug levels need to be kept at the therapeutic level using a _____.

a. loading dose
b. maintenance dose
c. toxic dose
d. lethal dose
e. local effect

DOSAGE CALCULATIONS (5)

1. What is the therapeutic index if the TD_{50} is 70 and ED_{50} is 10?

2. If the therapeutic index is 10 and the ED_{50} is 20, what is the TD_{50}?

3. What is the ED_{50} when TD_{50} is 150 and the therapeutic index is 20?

4. For Drug A, TD_{50} is 80 and ED_{50} is 10. For Drug B, the TD_{50} is 200 and ED_{50} is 50. Based on the therapeutic index of Drug A and Drug B, which one is safer?

5. For Drug C, the TD_{50} is 100 and ED_{50} is 20. For Drug D, the TD_{50} is 90 and ED_{50} is 30. Based on the therapeutic index of Drug C and Drug D, which one is more dangerous?

VISUAL CRITICAL THINKING (6)

1. Place the words *animals & fungi, genetically engineered, minerals, plants,* and *synthetic* in the correct category sources of drugs.

Sources of Drugs

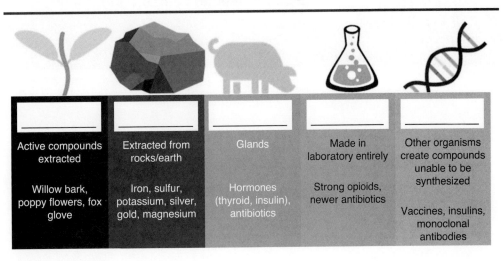

Active compounds extracted	Extracted from rocks/earth	Glands	Made in laboratory entirely	Other organisms create compounds unable to be synthesized
Willow bark, poppy flowers, fox glove	Iron, sulfur, potassium, silver, gold, magnesium	Hormones (thyroid, insulin), antibiotics	Strong opioids, newer antibiotics	Vaccines, insulins, monoclonal antibodies

Chapter **2** **Drug Actions (Pharmacodynamics)**

2. Place the correct definitions (limited to administration site, widespread through the body) and types of effects (local, systemic) with the proper drug effects.

Drug effects

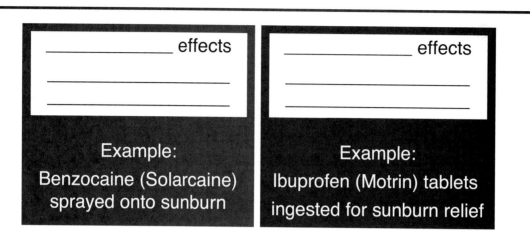

3. Place the correct type of dose (lethal, loading, maintenance, toxic) in the diagram matching its definition.

Dosing levels

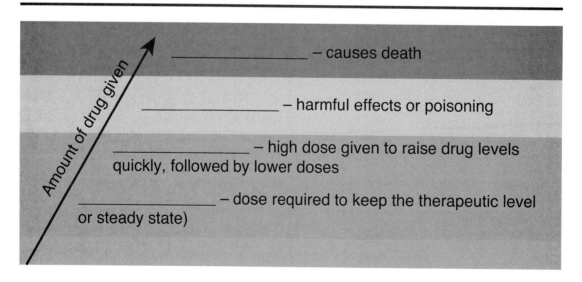

4. Place the terms *high* and *low* in the diagram.

Receptors

_____ affinity: will stick and stay at receptor for a while

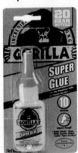

_____ affinity: will attach to receptor but can switch quickly

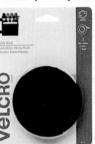

5. Place the correct terms, *narrow* and *wide*, matching the definition in the diagram.

Therapeutic index

- A _____ therapeutic index means they have a small window of safe doses

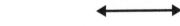

- A _____ therapeutic index is the opposite in that they have a larger window of safe doses

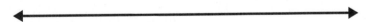

- Drugs with a narrow therapeutic index need to be dosed carefully and monitored frequently by pharmacists and doctors

6. Place TD_{50} and ED_{50} correctly in the equation and on the graph.

Therapeutic index

- Therapeutic index is the window of drug doses that can be used in patients that are both efficacious and non-lethal
- You can calculate the therapeutic index yourself!

Therapeutic index $= \dfrac{\boxed{}}{\boxed{}}$

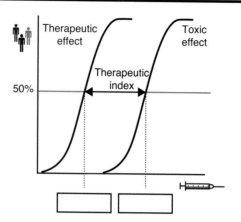

3 Drug Movement (Pharmacokinetics)

TRUE FALSE (10)

1. Pharmacokinetics is the study of drug movements throughout the body. _____
2. Distribution is when a drug is altered chemically within the body. _____
3. Catabolism is the breakdown of molecules into smaller parts. _____
4. The distribution of a drug is poor when a patient takes medication with food and it delays stomach emptying. _____
5. Chronic kidney disease affects the excretion of a drug, so we need to lower the dosage or increase the time interval between doses. _____
6. When a drug is fat-soluble, it can stay in the blood and spaces between the cells. _____
7. How quickly or slowly the body breaks the drug down is called "dissolving." _____
8. Most absorption occurs in the stomach. _____
9. A typical target for drugs is fat tissue because it makes the drug stay longer in the body. _____
10. We generally give patients with kidney disease the regular dose because it will remain at safe levels. _____

MULTIPLE CHOICE (10)

1. When a drug stays in the body longer, it is because of changes in _____.
   a. absorption
   b. distribution
   c. metabolism
   d. excretion

2. While dissolution is how fast a drug comes out of a vehicle, we consider how quickly or slowly the body breaks down a drug into smaller parts as _____.
   a. distributing
   b. dissolving
   c. absorbing
   d. excreting

3. All are part of the pharmacokinetic components *except*:
   a. absorption.
   b. dissolution.
   c. excretion.
   d. metabolism.

4. Metabolism involves which processes? *(Select all that apply.)*
   a. embolism
   b. anabolism
   c. constructivism
   d. catabolism

5. When a patient takes medication, the role of the stomach is _____, which helps the _____.
   a. breaking down the drug well enough; small intestine do its work
   b. absorbing the drug thoroughly; large intestine do its work
   c. excreting the drug out of the body; kidneys do their work
   d. distributing the drug throughout the body; blood vessels do their work

6. When a patient takes medication for asthma through an inhaler, this is an example of a(n) _____.
   a. inflammatory effect
   b. toxic effect
   c. localized effect
   d. systemic effect

7. For older adult patients, the prescriber needs to consider drugs that are not _____-soluble.
   a. water
   b. lipid
   c. enteric
   d. chemically

8. For a drug to stay in the body longer, a common target is _____ tissue.
   a. epithelial
   b. muscle
   c. adipose
   d. connective

9. It is important to know drugs will change into _____ because _____.
   a. active drugs; they can change the genetic sequence of the body
   b. smaller molecules; they can be excreted at a faster rate
   c. other drugs; they can initiate a therapeutic effect
   d. metabolites; it is crucial to administer the drugs safely

10. Some factors that negatively affect metabolism are: *(Select all that apply.)*
    a. disease.
    b. impaired organ function.
    c. race.
    d. mental state.

MATCHING (5)

Match the pharmacokinetic process to its description.

1. _____ Also known as destructive metabolism, in which the body breaks molecules apart
2. _____ A drug absorbed into the body
3. _____ The body removes a drug from the body
4. _____ Also known as constructive metabolism, in which the body synthesizes molecules
5. _____ Drug moves into intracellular spaces and extracellular spaces

a. absorption
b. distribution
c. excretion
d. catabolism
e. anabolism

COMPLETION (5)

1. _____ is how fast a drug comes out of a capsule.

2. The process of _____ is how quickly or slowly the body breaks a drug down into smaller components.

3. Whether a drug is water-soluble or lipid-soluble can affect the _____.

4. Metabolism is a process that is involved in _____.

5. Studying how the drug affects the body is called _____.

a. pharmacokinetics
b. pharmacodynamics
c. dissolution
d. dissolving
e. distribution

DOSAGE CALCULATIONS (5)

1. If a drug is 500 mg, two half-lives will reduce the drug to how many milligrams?

2. A drug level went from 1000 mg to 125 mg in the body. How many half-lives did this drug undergo?

3. A patient takes a drug that is 200 mg with a half-life of 1 hour. How much drug in milligrams remains after 4 hours?

4. A doctor prescribes a patient a drug that is 500 mg, taken once a day and has a half-life of 12 hours. The patient must take it for three days. After three days, how many half-lives in total have occurred?

5. A 1200 mg drug has a half-life of 2 hours. The patient took the pill at 7:00 am. At what time will 37.5 mg remain?

VISUAL CRITICAL THINKING (7)

1. Place the words *drug, motion,* and *movement* in the correct places.

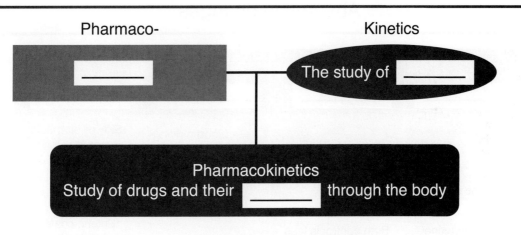

Definition – pharmacokinetics

Pharmaco-   Kinetics

The study of _____

Pharmacokinetics
Study of drugs and their _____ through the body

"What the body does to the drug"

2. Place the words *absorption, distribution, excretion,* and *metabolism* above the correct description of the pharmacokinetic process.

Kinetics and ADME

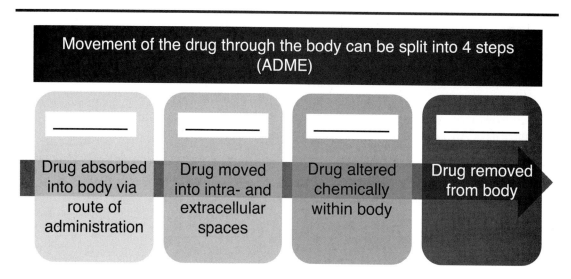

Movement of the drug through the body can be split into 4 steps (ADME)			
_____	_____	_____	_____
Drug absorbed into body via route of administration	Drug moved into intra- and extracellular spaces	Drug altered chemically within body	Drug removed from body

3. Place the words *age, blood flow, food,* and *illness,* to match the correct absorption change.

Absorption changes

_____	Gastrointestinal _____	_____	_____
Delays stomach emptying	Passage through GI tract speeds up (loose stools, diarrhea)	Less blood moving around small intestine allows less drug absorption	Slower stomach emptying, less breaking down of medications (dissolution)
Levothyroxine needs empty stomach	Birth control is less effective with antibiotics and illness	All drugs become less effective	Enteric-coated aspirin is released sooner, causing more GI adverse drug reactions

4. Place the words *adipose* and *hemodynamic* to match the correct distribution change.

Distribution changes

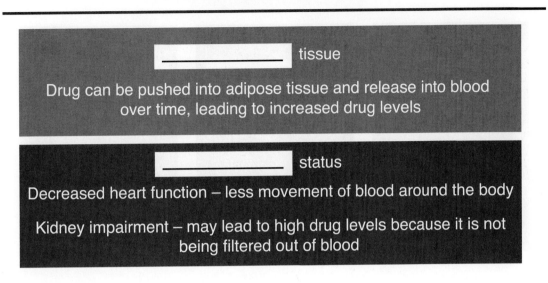

_____ tissue

Drug can be pushed into adipose tissue and release into blood over time, leading to increased drug levels

_____ status

Decreased heart function – less movement of blood around the body

Kidney impairment – may lead to high drug levels because it is not being filtered out of blood

5. Place the words *antibiotic, bacteria, bladder,* and *metabolism* to match the correct metabolism change.

Metabolism

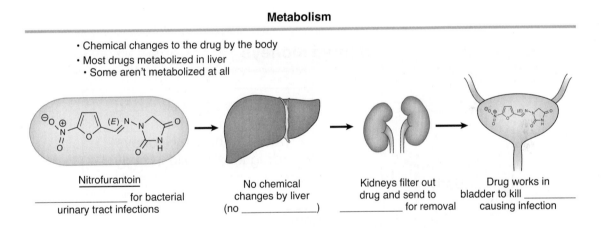

• Chemical changes to the drug by the body
• Most drugs metabolized in liver
• Some aren't metabolized at all

Nitrofurantoin

_____ for bacterial
urinary tract infections

No chemical
changes by liver
(no _____)

Kidneys filter out
drug and send to
_____ for removal

Drug works in
bladder to kill _____
causing infection

Chapter **3**   **Drug Movement (Pharmacokinetics)**

6. Place the terms *chronic kidney disease, dehydration,* and *hypotension* above the correct process of excretion changes.

Causes for excretion changes

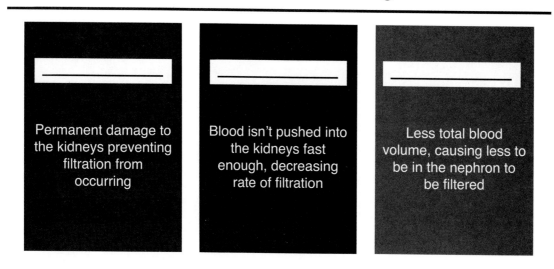

| _____ | _____ | _____ |
| Permanent damage to the kidneys preventing filtration from occurring | Blood isn't pushed into the kidneys fast enough, decreasing rate of filtration | Less total blood volume, causing less to be in the nephron to be filtered |

7. Place the terms *injured* and *slower* in the figure.

Injured kidneys

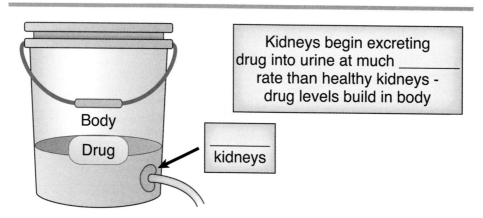

Body

Drug

_____ kidneys

Kidneys begin excreting drug into urine at much _____ rate than healthy kidneys - drug levels build in body

4 Drug Laws and Preventing Medication Errors

TRUE FALSE (10)

1. The Drug Enforcement Administration is a branch of the United States Department of Health and Human Services. _____

2. Food and Drug Administration (FDA) responsibilities include the management of cosmetics, medicines, medical devices, and bottled water. _____

3. The Centers for Disease Control and Prevention (CDC) enforces controlled substance laws and regulations and prosecutes those who grow and manufacture illegal substances. _____

4. Usually, state laws are stricter than federal regulations. _____

5. The Pure Food and Drug Act created the DEA. _____

6. Examples of Schedule IV drugs are benzodiazepines and Ambien, which have a low potential for abuse or dependence. _____

7. The sulfanilamide elixir tragedy led to the creation of the Pure Food and Drug Act. _____

8. NSAIDs can cause ulceration. _____

9. HIPAA allows healthcare providers to disclose health information for treatment or payment. _____

10. Tall man letters can reduce the medication errors in drugs that look alike or sound alike. _____

MULTIPLE CHOICE (10)

1. Which agency is a branch of the United States Department of Health and Human Services?
   a. Centers for Disease Control and Prevention (CDC)
   b. Food and Drug Administration (FDA)
   c. Department of Justice (DOJ)
   d. Drug Enforcement Administration (DEA)

2. Which federal acts or amendments required manufacturers to prove that a drug was safe as part of a new drug application before marketing and sale?
   a. Pure Food and Drug Act of 1906
   b. Durham-Humphrey Amendment of 1951
   c. Food, Drug, and Cosmetic Act of 1938
   d. Comprehensive Drug Abuse Prevention and Control Act of 1970

3. The Durham-Humphrey Amendment of 1951 states that:
   a. manufacturers must prove that a drug is safe as part of a new drug application before marketing and sale.
   b. the Food and Drug Administration also manages potentially addictive medications.
   c. manufacturers must report side effects that occurred after approval.
   d. the Food and Drug Administration has the authority to determine whether medications are safe to use without a prescription, over the counter, or if they require a prescription.

4. Which are *not* Schedule II drugs? *(Select all that apply.)*
   a. heroin
   b. morphine
   c. pregabalin
   d. amphetamines

5. Drugs such as diphenoxylate atropine and cough syrups with limited amounts of codeine have:
   a. the lowest potential for abuse or dependence.
   b. high potential for abuse and have an accepted medical use.
   c. low potential for abuse or dependence.
   d. high potential for abuse and no accepted medical use.

6. What criteria determine if a package is child-resistant? *(Select all that apply.)*
   a. 80% of adults can open the package
   b. 90% of children younger than 5 years cannot open the package
   c. 90% of adults can open the package
   d. 80% of children 5 years old cannot open the package

7. The Orphan Drug Act of 1983 was created to increase the treatment options for:
   a. genetic diseases only.
   b. rare diseases only.
   c. common diseases like the common cold only.
   d. children only.

8. HIPAA stands for:
   a. Health Insurance Protections and Accreditation Act.
   b. Health Information Portability and Accountability Act.
   c. Health Information Protections and Accreditation Act.
   d. Health Insurance Portability and Accountability Act.

9. Which drug ingredients are regulated through the Combat Methamphetamine Epidemic Act of 2005? *(Select all that apply.)*
   a. ephedrine
   b. cocaine
   c. pseudoephedrine
   d. phenylpropanolamine

10. Which can help reduce medication errors due to look-alike sound-alike drugs? *(Select all that apply.)*
    a. Using child-resistance packaging
    b. Using tall man letters
    c. Using brand and generic names on labels
    d. Using same color medication bottle

MATCHING (5)

Match the drug to the corresponding drug schedule.

1. _____ ketamine
2. _____ ecstasy
3. _____ morphine
4. _____ diphenoxylate/atropine
5. _____ benzodiazepine

a. Schedule I
b. Schedule II
c. Schedule III
d. Schedule IV
e. Schedule V

COMPLETION (5)

1. The country enacted the _____ as a result of the sulfanilamide elixir tragedy.

2. The Thalidomide Disaster of 1962 led to the creation of the _____, which increased regulation of drugs that can be on the market.

3. Drug schedules were created after Congress passed the _____.

4. Due to children taking pills that looked like candy, the _____ passed, which gave the Consumer Product Safety Commission power to establish standards for drug packaging.

5. The _____ helps increase treatment options for a rare disease that affects fewer than 200,000 people.
   a. Kefauver Harris Amendment
   b. Food, Drug, and Cosmetic Act (FDCA) of 1938
   c. Orphan Drug Act of 1983
   d. Poison Prevention Packaging Act of 1970
   e. Comprehensive Drug Abuse Prevention and Control Act of 1970

DOSAGE CALCULATIONS (5)

1. In Iowa, a person bought 30 g of pseudoephedrine in a year. How many months' worth of pseudoephedrine did they purchase?

2. Under federal law, if a person can purchase 9 g of pseudoephedrine per month in 2 years, what is the maximum amount in grams they can buy in that period?

3. A patient purchased a total of 54 g of pseudoephedrine. Under federal law, this equates to how many months' worth of pseudoephedrine?

4. If a state only allowed 8 g of pseudoephedrine to be purchased per month, how much total would be allowed for 3 months?

5. A patient purchased pseudoephedrine in a state that allows the purchase of only 6.5 g of pseudoephedrine per month. They went to Pharmacy A, bought 13 g of pseudoephedrine, and then bought 39 g of pseudoephedrine at Pharmacy B. How many full months' worth of pseudoephedrine did they buy?

VISUAL CRITICAL THINKING (3)

1. What type of drug did this image represent?

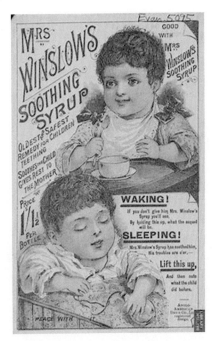

Chapter **4** **Drug Laws and Preventing Medication Errors**

2. What is an essential component of packaging drugs and other household products to prevent poisoning?

3. What is the critical federal act/amendment to address the problem of children trying to get into medication bottles?

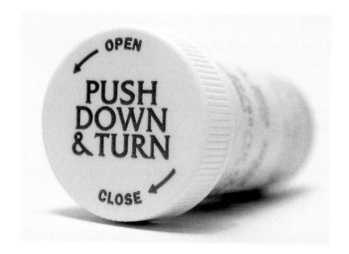

5 Drug Administration

TRUE FALSE (10)

1. One example of the enteral route is gastrostomy. _____
2. A parenteral medication goes through the GI tract. _____
3. A tablet is a solid dosage form that can be given orally. _____
4. A suspension is clear with the drug wholly dissolved. _____
5. The buccal route can skip the first-pass effect. _____
6. Enteral administration must be aseptic. _____
7. The gauge of the needle is the shaft's diameter. _____
8. The syringe has three parts: the bevel, hub, and shaft. _____
9. Intradermal is an example of parenteral administration. _____
10. Ophthalmic drops are sometimes prescribed for an ear infection, which can also be used in the eye. _____

MULTIPLE CHOICE (10)

1. Which are enteral forms? *(Select all that apply.)*
   a. sublingual
   b. subcutaneous
   c. nasogastric
   d. rectal

2. For the oral route of administration, some common dosage forms are: *(Select all that apply.)*
   a. intramuscular.
   b. tablet.
   c. capsule.
   d. lozenge.

3. Which is a liquid dosage form if a liquid is not an equal mixture with another?
   a. emulsion
   b. elixir
   c. syrup
   d. suspension

4. The benefit of using the _____ dosage form is that there is direct absorption into the circulation and the first-pass effect does not occur.
   a. nasojejunal
   b. nasogastric
   c. oral
   d. sublingual

5. What dosage form would be most appropriate for an unconscious patient?
   a. solution
   b. emulsion
   c. intravenous
   d. sublingual

6. An intramuscular injection is given at a _____-degree angle.
   a. 30
   b. 45
   c. 60
   d. 90

7. An intramuscular (IM) injection goes directly _____.
   a. into the subarachnoid space of the spine
   b. into the muscle
   c. under the skin
   d. on top layers of the skin

8. For an inhalation route of administration, which is/are the most appropriate dosage form(s)? *(Select all that apply.)*
   a. gas
   b. vapor
   c. suspension
   d. powder

9. Ophthalmic drops can be used in the _____. *(Select all that apply.)*
   a. ear
   b. eyes
   c. nose
   d. mouth

10. A needle has _____ parts: the _____.
    a. 3; plunger, tip, and barrel
    b. 4; plunger, shaft, barrel, and tip
    c. 3; bevel, hub, and cannula
    d. 4; hub, barrel, tip, and plunger

MATCHING (5)

Match the administration method to the description.

1. _____ subcutaneous
2. _____ intravenous
3. _____ intramuscular
4. _____ intrathecal
5. _____ intradermal

a. into the vein
b. into the skin
c. below the skin
d. into the muscle
e. into the spinal canal

COMPLETION (5)

1. The _____ is used when a patient has an eye infection, irritation, or allergy.

2. Smoking cessation can be provided through the _____.

3. To avoid systemic effects, the _____ is used for sinuses.

4. Asthma medications are often used through the _____ to target the organ that is affected, such as the lungs.

5. Medications that require the _____ can go directly into the ear canal but cannot go into the eye.

a. transdermal route
b. ophthalmic route
c. nasal route
d. otic route
e. inhalation route

DOSAGE CALCULATIONS (5)

1. A patient has to take two 5-mg tablets twice a day for 7 days. How many total milligrams does this patient have to take?

2. Nitroglycerin is often given sublingually to bypass the first-pass effect. First-pass metabolism clears 90% of a nitroglycerin capsule of 3 mg. How much of the nitroglycerin capsule in milligrams is removed from the body?

3. The pharmacy has three 5-mL vials of the flu vaccine left. Each patient is given 0.5 mL of the vaccine. How many patients can receive flu shots?

4. A patient needs to take one 21-mg nicotine patch per day every day for 4 weeks. How many patches would they need in total?

5. A patient took two sprays in each nostril for allergies once a day for 5 days and one spray in each nostril once a day for 2 days. Each spray is 55 mcg. How many micrograms in total did the patient spray?

VISUAL CRITICAL THINKING (7)

Fill in the blanks on the figures.

1. Nasogastric and gastrostomy. Place the terms *esophagus, nasogastric,* and *stomach* in the figure.

Nasogastric and Gastrostomy

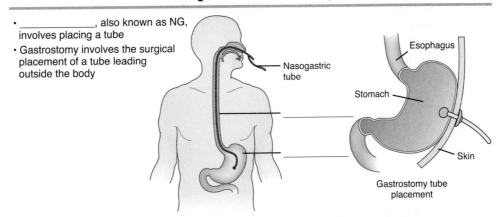

- _____, also known as NG, involves placing a tube
- Gastrostomy involves the surgical placement of a tube leading outside the body

Nasogastric tube

Esophagus

Stomach

Skin

Gastrostomy tube placement

2. Sublingual. Place the terms *nauseous, nitroglycerin, ondansetron,* and *quick* in the figure.

Sublingual

- An advantage of the sublingual route is that the onset is _____ and avoids the stomach and first-pass effect
- Great for _____ patients as well
- May cause some irritation of the mouth
- Medication examples include:
  - _____ for nausea
  - _____ for chest pain

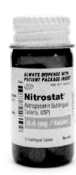

3. Parenteral administration – equipment. Place the terms *bevel, hub, lumen,* and *shaft* in the figure.

Parenteral adminstration – equipment

- Needles are made up of three parts: <u>bevel</u>, <u>cannula</u>, and <u>hub</u>
  - Bevel: slanted part at the needle's tip
  - Cannula: actual metal part of needle
  - Hub: part of the needle that connects into the syringe

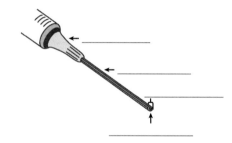

4. Intravenous: Place the words *into the veins* and *25 degrees* in the correct place.

Intravenous

- The intravenous route involves administering medications _____
  - This provides direct access to the circulation
- Injecting intravenously uses an angle of _____
- The intravenous route is the most common administration route, and the majority of medications are given this way in the hospital

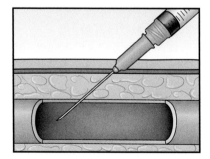

5. Subcutaneous. Place the terms *45, fatty,* and *skin* into the figure.

Subcutaneous

- The subcutaneous route requires injecting the medication into the _____ tissue under the _____
- The angle or subcutaneous injection is _____ degrees
- A common medication given subcutaneously is insulin

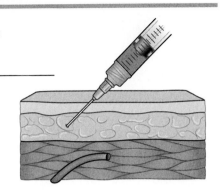

6. Intramuscular. Place the terms *90* and *skeletal* into the figure.

Intramuscular

- An intramuscular injection is just how it sounds, you inject medications into the _____ muscle
- The angle for intramuscular administration is _____ degrees
- A common medication given intramuscularly is flu the shot, given every Fall

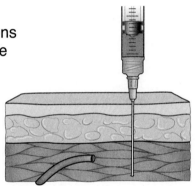

7. Intrathecal. Place the terms *baclofen, palsy, spine,* and *sterile* into the figure.

Intrathecal

- Intrathecal administration involves giving the medication into the subarachnoid space of the _____
- This process must be _____ as bacteria getting into the spinal fluid can be deadly
- An example of a medication given intrathecally is _____ for cerebral _____

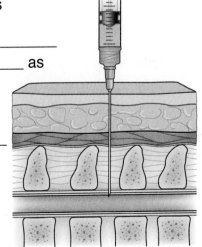

6 Dosage Calculations

TRUE FALSE (10)

1. A microgram is 1/1000 of a gram. _____
2. A milliequivalent is where a milligram equivalent is listed next to the number of milliequivalents. _____
3. The ratio and proportion method is also known as the desired-over-have method. _____
4. The factor-label method is another name for the dimensional analysis method. _____
5. Ten cubic centimeters is equal to 100 mL. _____
6. Five teaspoons are equivalent to 25 milliliters. _____
7. Cubic centimeters are a measurement of weight. _____
8. To convert pounds to kg, you need to use (1 kg/2.2 lbs) as a conversion factor. _____
9. An accurate method to measure liquid medication can be done with any kitchen spoon. _____
10. Plastic syringes are more accurate to ensure that the proper dosage is given. _____

MULTIPLE CHOICE (10)

1. Which are measures of weight? *(Select all that apply.)*
   a. gram
   b. micrograms
   c. milliequivalent
   d. liter

2. The abbreviation "cc" is a measure of _____, which stands for cubic _____.
   a. weight; centimeter
   b. volume; centiliter
   c. volume; centimeter
   d. weight; centiliter

3. A patient needs to take 600 mg in total. The prescription states to take one 100-mg tablet twice a day by mouth. How many pills does the pharmacy need to dispense?
   a. Two tablets
   b. Four tablets
   c. Six tablets
   d. Eight tablets

4. A medication bottle contains 135 mL of liquid acetaminophen. The directions say to take 30 mL every night. How many tablespoons total can be taken?
   a. Six tablespoons
   b. Seven tablespoons
   c. Eight tablespoons
   d. Nine tablespoons

5. For liquid acetaminophen, there is a total of 120 mg in 10 mL. A patient needs to receive a 5-mL dose. The conversion factor _____ should be used to determine that a patient needs to receive _____ mg of medication.
   a. 120 mg / 15 mL; 40
   b. 120 mg / 20 mL; 30
   c. 120 mg / 10 mL; 60
   d. 120 mg/ 5 mL; 120

6. A _____ is one kilogram of water in standard conditions.
   a. milliliter
   b. teaspoon
   c. tablespoon
   d. liter

7. A nurse requires 1 L of IV saline bag solution. How many mL are in the IV saline bag solution?
   a. 10 mL
   b. 100 mL
   c. 1000 mL
   d. 10,000 mL

8. When a liquid medication is dispensed, it is vital to include a _____. *(Select all that apply.)*
   a. measuring cup
   b. conversion instructions
   c. plastic syringe
   d. metal kitchen spoon

9. What methods of calculation can be used? *(Select all that apply.)*
   a. ratio and proportion method
   b. formula method
   c. dimensional analysis method
   d. standard fraction deviation

10. The pound (lb) is equal to _____ kilograms.
    a. 0.5576
    b. 0.6546
    c. 0.4536
    d. 0.5546

MATCHING (5)

Match the volume measurement to its equivalence conversion.

1. _____ teaspoon
2. _____ tablespoon
3. _____ cubic centimeter
4. _____ milliliter
5. _____ fluid ounce

a. equal to 1 milliliter
b. equal to 5 milliliters
c. equal to 15 milliliters
d. equal to 30 milliliters
e. 0.001 of a liter

COMPLETION (5)

1. _____ is used as an equation that says two fractions across from each other are equivalent.

2. Also known as the unit-factor method, the _____ can change one quantity to another.

3. Factors can be converted with _____ by knowing the ordered dose, the amount on hand, and the medicine quantity.

4. The kilogram is the base mass unit in the metric system, also known as the _____.

5. An example of _____ is milligrams per hour, which is a comparison in fraction form.

a. ratio
b. formula method
c. dimensional analysis method
d. proportion
e. international system of units

DOSAGE CALCULATIONS (5)

1. If a patient needs 1000 mg of medication and there are 200 mg in each tablet, how many tablets would the patient need to take?

2. A child weighs 50 pounds. How much does this child weigh in kilograms?

3. Acetaminophen is dosed at 5 mg/kg. How much acetaminophen can a 77-pound child receive?

4. A child needs to receive 30 mL of a 150 mg/10 mL drug. How much in milligrams should be given to the child?

5. A patient's prescription instructs the patient to take two 50-mg tablets once a day for 2 weeks. How much will the total dosage be in milligrams?

VISUAL CRITICAL THINKING (7)

1. Describe why using a regular metal kitchen spoon is inappropriate.

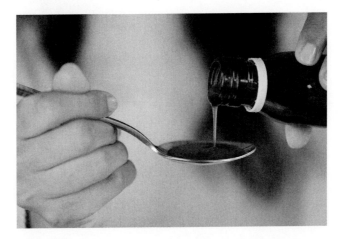

2. What would you recommend to a parent whose child does not want to take chewable cold medication because they don't like how it tastes?

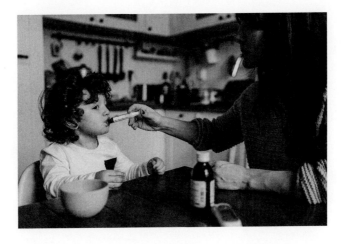

3. Why does a measuring cup or measuring syringe provide a more accurate dose?

4. What else should be included when dispensing a liquid medication?

5. What would you recommend to a parent who calls about how many times they should give their child 2.5 mL of liquid medication using a 5-mL measuring cup?

6. Describe how to respond to a parent's concern about giving medication using a plastic syringe to their child because it reminds them of when they get immunization shots at the doctor's office.

7. State the unit of measurement used in measuring cups or a plastic syringe.

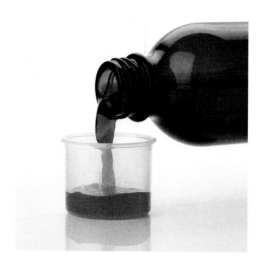

7 Drug Classifications

TRUE FALSE (10)

1. NSAID drugs have a *-cillin* suffix. _____
2. Generic names can come from the physical structure. _____
3. Common drugs used to treat acid reflux end in *-tidine*. _____
4. Proton pump inhibitors are available both over the counter (OTC) and by prescription. _____
5. Opioid analgesics are related to methylprednisolone. _____
6. Bisphosphonates are often used for patients whose bones have become weaker. _____
7. Bronchodilators can help open up the bronchioles in asthma. _____
8. Expectorants are medications that can help prevent a cough. _____
9. Prevnar-13 is a vaccine that can prevent a fungal infection. _____
10. Patients with Parkinson's disease may be prescribed Sinemet, which helps activate dopamine. _____

MULTIPLE CHOICE (10)

1. Which are antianxiety medications? *(Select all that apply.)*
   a. midazolam
   b. lorazepam
   c. levodopa/carbidopa
   d. eletriptan

2. When a generic medication name has *pred-* in its name, this generally indicates that it is a(n):
   a. opioid.
   b. proton pump inhibitor.
   c. steroid.
   d. beta-blocker.

3. Histamine-2 receptor antagonists are used for _____ and histamine-1 receptor antagonists are used for _____.
   a. seasonal allergies; heart failure
   b. heart failure; seasonal allergies
   c. seasonal allergies; heartburn
   d. heartburn; seasonal allergies

4. The suffix *-prazole* is a stem for which drug class?
   a. proton pump inhibitors
   b. antipsychotics
   c. histamine-2 receptor antagonists
   d. bisphosphonates

5. While all of the following are for pain, which are considered narcotic analgesics? *(Select all that apply.)*
   a. hydrocodone/acetaminophen
   b. ibuprofen
   c. celecoxib
   d. oxycodone/acetaminophen

6. To treat asthma, _____ helps open up the bronchioles and _____ helps prevent the inflammation.
   a. fluticasone; albuterol
   b. albuterol; fluticasone
   c. budesonide; albuterol
   d. budesonide; ipratropium

7. Which treats bacterial infection?
   a. azithromycin
   b. acyclovir
   c. valacyclovir
   d. fluconazole

8. Which drug works to provide relief for patients with Parkinson's disease?
   a. amitriptyline
   b. sertraline
   c. sumatriptan
   d. levodopa/carbidopa

9. A physician prescribes a second-generation drug for a patient with schizophrenia because of the first-generation drug's adverse effects. Which could the physician prescribe? *(Select all that apply.)*
   a. Thorazine
   b. Zyprexa
   c. Rexulti
   d. Abilify

10. Which drug is considered an angiotensin II receptor blocker?
    a. Zestril
    b. Cozaar
    c. Lotensin
    d. Inderal

MATCHING (5)

Match the medication to the drug class.

1. _____ Prozac
2. _____ Tagamet
3. _____ Mucinex
4. _____ Effexor
5. _____ Remicade

a. expectorant
b. histamine-2 receptor antagonist
c. monoclonal antibody
d. selective serotonin reuptake inhibitor
e. serotonin-norepinephrine reuptake inhibitor

COMPLETION (5)

1. _____ is a second-generation drug for schizophrenia.

2. As a serotonin receptor agonist, _____ is a medication that can help with migraines.

3. Benzodiazepines such as _____ help induce sleep and reduce anxiety.

4. _____ is a common analgesic medication used to avoid gastrointestinal-related side effects.

5. A medication like _____ can help patients with heart failure.

a. midazolam
b. furosemide
c. eletriptan
d. olanzapine
e. celecoxib

1. Review the following list of medications: famotidine, nizatidine, aripiprazole, and brexpiprazole. How many are histamine-2 receptor antagonists and proton pump inhibitors?

2. Based on the brand names in this list: Advil, Motrin, Naprosyn, Tylenol, Celebrex, how many are NSAIDs?

3. How many prescription medications are dispensed based on the following prescription list: Advair, Tylenol, Xanax, and Mucinex?

4. Out of these drugs: loratadine, pseudoephedrine, oxymetazoline, cetirizine, and guaifenesin, how many can be used as antihistamines only?

5. Based on this list's generic names: alprazolam, lorazepam, clonazepam, and carbamazepine, which ones are considered benzodiazepines?

8 | Gastrointestinal

TRUE FALSE (10)

1. A pH of 2 would be acidic, rather than basic. _____
2. Bismuth subsalicylate is safe for children. _____
3. Calcium carbonate is a proton pump inhibitor (PPI). _____
4. Diphenoxylate/atropine is a controlled substance. _____
5. *Helicobacter pylori* is a gram-positive bacterium. _____
6. Loperamide is an example of an antacid. _____
7. Promethazine affects the chemoreceptor trigger zone (CTZ). _____
8. Psyllium is a bulk-forming laxative. _____
9. The "S" form, such as esomeprazole, is more biologically active. _____
10. The stem identifying famotidine as an H_2 blocker is *-tidine*. _____

MULTIPLE CHOICE (10)

1. A medication that ends in *-prazole* is most likely a(n):
   a. antiemetic.
   b. PPI.
   c. H_2 receptor antagonist (H2RA).
   d. laxative.

2. A patient who needs an over-the-counter (OTC) PPI should use:
   a. calcium carbonate (Tums).
   b. magnesium hydroxide (Milk of Magnesia).
   c. esomeprazole (Nexium).
   d. famotidine (Pepcid).

3. Calcium carbonate would be classified as a(n):
   a. bulk-forming laxative.
   b. antacid.
   c. stool softener.
   d. H2RA.

4. Someone looking for an antidiarrheal would use which medication?
   a. esomeprazole (Nexium)
   b. famotidine (Pepcid)
   c. loperamide (Imodium)
   d. polyethylene glycol (MiraLAX)

5. Which is scheduled by the DEA?
   a. diphenoxylate/atropine (Lomotil)
   b. omeprazole (Prilosec)
   c. loperamide (Imodium)
   d. polyethylene glycol (MiraLAX)

6. All of the following medicines would be appropriate for constipation *except*:
   a. docusate (Colace).
   b. psyllium (Metamucil).
   c. famotidine (Pepcid).
   d. polyethylene glycol (MiraLAX).

7. Patients should know that magnesium sulfate (Milk of Magnesia) can cause which side effect?
   a. constipation
   b. black tongue and stools
   c. diarrhea
   d. acid reflux

8. Which is a common side effect of calcium carbonate (Tums)?
   a. constipation
   b. headache
   c. dizziness
   d. diarrhea

9. Which is the correct mechanism of action for acid-reducer omeprazole (Prilosec)?
   a. activates histamine receptors
   b. 5-HT3 antagonist
   c. blocks histamine receptors
   d. inhibits proton pumps

10. Famotidine is in which drug class?
    a. laxative
    b. H2RA
    c. antibiotic
    d. immunomodulator

MATCHING (5)

Match the medication to the drug class.

1. _____ omeprazole
2. _____ famotidine
3. _____ psyllium
4. _____ loperamide
5. _____ infliximab

a. antidiarrheal
b. H2RA
c. immunomodulator
d. laxative
e. PPI

COMPLETION (5)

1. _____ is an H2RA for acid reduction.

2. If a patient needed an antacid, they might rely on _____.

3. Only _____ would help with diarrhea.

4. To prevent proton pumps from working, a patient might use _____.

5. We could classify _____ as a stool softener.

a. calcium carbonate
b. docusate sodium
c. omeprazole
d. loperamide
e. famotidine

DOSAGE CALCULATIONS (5)

1. If a patient cannot take more than 360 mg of omeprazole in a day, how many capsules would the maximum be if the capsules are 20 mg each?

2. When calculating a dose for treating an ulcer, we often see a PPI like esomeprazole used once daily for 10 days. However, the patient needs 40 mg per day and we only have 20-mg capsules. How many total capsules will the patient need?

3. If a 12-year-old child is to get 20 mg once a day for 4 weeks, how many milligrams did they take over the span of the treatment?

4. A 22-pound child needs 0.5 mg/kg/day of famotidine at bedtime. How many milligrams does the patient need in each daily dose?

5. A patient is told to take two 2-mg loperamide tablets at the outset of diarrhea symptoms and one tablet with each additional movement, but not to take more than four tablets in 24 hours. What is the maximum daily dose in milligrams?

VISUAL CRITICAL THINKING (5)

Fill in the missing words in the figures below.

1. PUD causes (invaders). Place the terms *healing, mucus, negative,* and *prostaglandin* in the figure.

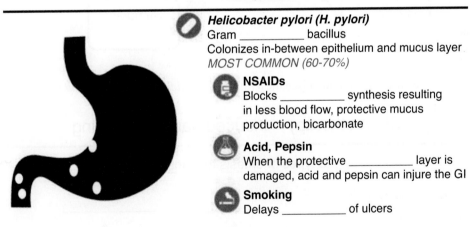

PUD Causes (Invaders)

Helicobacter pylori (H. pylori)
Gram _____ bacillus
Colonizes in-between epithelium and mucus layer
MOST COMMON (60-70%)

NSAIDs
Blocks _____ synthesis resulting in less blood flow, protective mucus production, bicarbonate

Acid, Pepsin
When the protective _____ layer is damaged, acid and pepsin can injure the GI

Smoking
Delays _____ of ulcers

2. PUD treatment – non-drug. Place the terms *alcohol, caffeine, meals, NSAIDs,* and *smoking* in the figure.

PUD treatment - *non-drug*

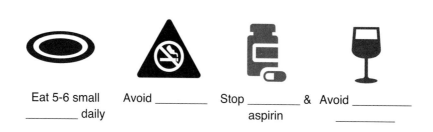

Eat 5-6 small _____ daily   Avoid _____   Stop _____ & aspirin   Avoid _____ _____

Last: reduce stress as much as possible

3. Constipation treatment – laxatives *(Fill in the blanks with either "mush" or "push".)*

Constipation treatment – laxatives

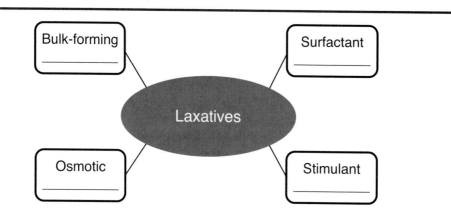

Bulk-forming
_____

Surfactant
_____

Laxatives

Osmotic
_____

Stimulant
_____

4. Chemotherapy–induced nausea/vomiting. Place the *terms acute, anticipatory,* and *delayed* in the figure.

Chemotherapy – induced nausea/vomiting

3 types of emesis to manage

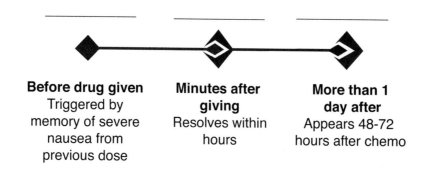

Before drug given
Triggered by memory of severe nausea from previous dose

Minutes after giving
Resolves within hours

More than 1 day after
Appears 48-72 hours after chemo

5. GI autoimmune pathology (IBD). Place the terms *Crohn disease* and *ulcerative colitis* in the figure.

GI Autoimmune Pathology (IBD)

Caused by exaggerated immune response to normal bowel flora

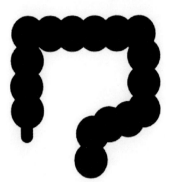

_____
- Inflammation of the mucosa and submucosa of the colon and rectum
- Can cause rectal bleeding
- May require hospitalization

_____
- Characterized by transmural inflammation
- Usually affects terminal ileum (can affect all parts of GI tract)

MNEMONICS (3)

1. Use the mnemonic ACIDIC MEALS to help you name four antacids and four side effects or interactions that concern you about antacids.

ACIDIC MEALS

A _____ (antacid)

C _____ (antacid)

I

D _____ P _____ (side effect)

I _____ C _____ (drug interaction)

C _____ (side effect)

M _____ (antacid)

E

A _____ N _____ (when / how to take antacids)

L _____ (side effect of magnesium hydroxide)

S _____ (antacid)

2. In order of aggressiveness of therapy from least to most, name three antidiarrheal or combination drugs. Use the mnemonic BUILD A BARRIER to help.

BUILD A BARRIER

B _____ (salicylate, least aggressive)

U

I

L _____ (opioid receptor agonist)

D _____ /

A _____ (opioid, anticholinergic combination, most aggressive)

BARRIER

39

3. In order of least to most aggressive treatment, name four drugs for constipation. Use the mnemonic PREDISPOSED to help you remember.

PREDISPOSED

P _____ (fiber)

R

E

D _____(stool softener)

I

S _____ (stimulant)

PO _____ G _____ (osmotic)

S

E

D

9 Musculoskeletal

TRUE FALSE (10)

1. Acetaminophen has the same cardiovascular benefits as aspirin. _____
2. ASA is a new medication for pain and inflammation. _____
3. Celecoxib is recommended for pregnant women. _____
4. Fentanyl is 100 times more potent than morphine. _____
5. Meloxicam has a longer duration of action than ibuprofen. _____
6. Miosis is a contraction of the pupils. _____
7. N-Acetyl-para-amino-phenol is a generic name. _____
8. NSAIDs can cause ulceration. _____
9. Opioids do not cause respiratory depression. _____
10. There are at least two COX enzymes involved with inflammation. _____

MULTIPLE CHOICE (10)

1. Which of the following are NSAIDs? *(Select all that apply.)*
    a. oxycodone (OxyContin)
    b. celecoxib (Celebrex)
    c. ibuprofen (Advil, Motrin)
    d. meloxicam (Mobic)

2. To which DEA schedule does tramadol belong?
    a. C - II
    b. C - III
    c. C - IV
    d. C - V

3. To which opioid side effect(s) would the patient develop tolerance? *(Select all that apply.)*
    a. analgesia
    b. constipation
    c. dizziness
    d. sedation

4. Which comes as a transdermal patch?
    a. fentanyl (Duragesic)
    b. morphine (MS Contin)
    c. naloxone (Narcan)
    d. tramadol (Ultram)

5. Which migraine medication(s) is/are best for prophylaxis? *(Select all that apply.)*
    a. amitriptyline (Elavil)
    b. ibuprofen (Advil, Motrin)
    c. propranolol (Inderal)
    d. sumatriptan (Imitrex)

6. Which medicine would one classify as a long-acting NSAID?
   a. acetaminophen (Tylenol)
   b. ibuprofen (Motrin, Advil)
   c. meloxicam (Mobic)
   d. methotrexate (Rheumatrex)

7. How would you define physical dependence?
   a. The dose increases, yet the patient gets the same response.
   b. The dose decreases and the patient gets the same response.
   c. A condition of possible withdrawal after the abrupt discontinuation of a medication.
   d. When the dose increases and the patient gets a heightened response.

8. Which is *not* an over-the-counter (OTC) medication?
   a. fentanyl (Duragesic)
   b. ibuprofen (Advil, Motrin)
   c. acetaminophen (Tylenol)
   d. naproxen (Aleve)

9. Which is/are DEA schedules? *(Select all that apply.)*
   a. C - VII
   b. C - II
   c. C - III
   d. C - X

10. What is the drug class of sumatriptan?
    a. 5-HT$_3$ agonist
    b. xanthine oxidase inhibitor
    c. NSAID
    d. DMARD

MATCHING (5)

Match the medication to the drug class.

1. _____ alendronate
2. _____ eletriptan
3. _____ ibuprofen
4. _____ methotrexate
5. _____ oxycodone

a. 5-HT receptor agonist
b. bisphosphonate
c. DMARD
d. NSAID
e. opioid analgesic

COMPLETION (5)

1. _____ is an NSAID for pain, fever, and inflammation.

2. If a patient had muscle spasms, they might rely on _____.

3. Only _____ would help with osteoporosis.

4. To prevent gout, a patient might use _____.

5. We could classify _____ as a biologic DMARD.

a. cyclobenzaprine
b. etanercept
c. febuxostat
d. ibandronate
e. naproxen

DOSAGE CALCULATIONS (5)

1. If a patient cannot take more than 3200 mg of ibuprofen in a day, how many tablets would the maximum be if the tablets are 200 mg each?

2. When calculating maximum acetaminophen doses, we must watch for multiple medications that include acetaminophen. If a patient takes hydrocodone/acetaminophen (Vicodin) three times in a day with 500 mg of acetaminophen in each tablet and one 650-mg extra-strength acetaminophen, how much acetaminophen did the patient take in a day?

3. A child weights 35 pounds and is supposed to get 2.5 mL of infant drops. How many milligrams does the child get if there are 50 mg in each 1.25 mL?

4. If there are 5 mL in a teaspoonful, and the patient has to take three teaspoonfuls of medication, how many mL do they need?

5. Children's acetaminophen (Tylenol) comes as 160 mg/5 mL and the 8-year-old patient is to take 10 mL. How many milligrams will the patient receive?

VISUAL CRITICAL THINKING (7)

1. Place the words *delta, kappa,* and *mu* to match the correct symbols.

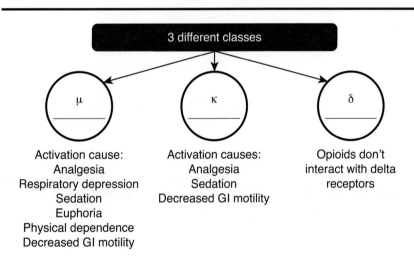

Opioid – receptors

3 different classes

μ

κ

δ

Activation cause:
Analgesia
Respiratory depression
Sedation
Euphoria
Physical dependence
Decreased GI motility

Activation causes:
Analgesia
Sedation
Decreased GI motility

Opioids don't
interact with delta
receptors

2. Place the following medications in their correct DEA class: ecstasy, fentanyl, testosterone, tramadol, Lomotil.

DEA schedules

All medications that work on opioid receptors are controlled substances C-I have no medical use and are illegal

Name	Schedule
Heroin, marijuana, _____	C-I
_____, oxycodone, Adderall, cocaine, hydrocodone	C-II
Acetaminophen/codeine, _____, anabolic steroids	C-III
_____, Xanax, Ativan, Ambien	C-IV
Cheratussin, _____, Lyrica	C-V

Abuse and dependence potential <u>decreases</u> as schedule number <u>increases</u>

3. Place the words *morphine, pinpoint,* and *pupillary* in the diagram.

Opioids - Morphine ADRs

Miosis

• _____ constriction
• Toxic doses: Pupils may constrict to "_____" size
  • Similar to pupils in bright lights
• Caused by _____ and other opioids

Triad symptom

4. Place *neural activation, neural trigger, signal amplification,* and *vasodilation & inflammation* in the correct order from 1 to 4.

Migraine – Pathology

Neurovascular disorder that involves dilation and inflammation of intracranial blood vessels

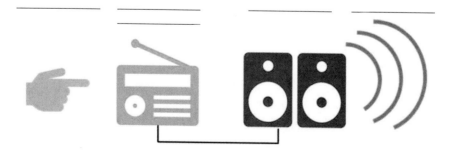

5. Place *5-hydroxytyptophan [5-HT] (serotonin)* and *calcitonin gene-related peptide (CGRP)* in the right positions on the see-saw.

Migraine – pathology

Two compounds thought to be at play:

_____
_____
- Promotes migraines
- Elevated during migraines

_____
_____
- Suppresses migraines
- Plasma levels drop during migraines
- Giving more 5-HT during migraine can abort it

6. Place *osteoblasts* and *osteoclasts* in the right positions.

Osteoporosis – Pathology

- Low bone mass and bone fragility
- Bone is the largest source of calcium in the body
- When body is low on calcium, _____ break down bone structure to free calcium
- _____ build bone structure back up, using calcium in circulation

Osteoids

7. Place *chronic, kings,* and *NSAIDs* in the correct positions.

Gout - Pathology

"The disease of _____"
- Buildup of uric acid, usually in big toe
  - Uric acid crystalize
  - Sharp, severe joint pain occurs
- _____ treatment involves decreasing uric acid levels
- _____ used as first-line, acute, flare-up treatment

1. Name eight DEA Schedule II opioids or opioid combinations. Use the mnemonic MY MY MY FREAKING HEAD HURTS OUCH OUCH to help you remember.

MY MY MY FREAKING HEAD HURTS OUCH OUCH

M _____ (opioid)

M _____ (opioid)

M _____ (opioid)

F _____ (opioid)

H _____ / A _____ (opioid / analgesic)

H _____ / I _____ (opioid / NSAID)

O _____ (opioid)

O _____ / A _____ (opioid / analgesic)

10 Respiratory

1. Diphenhydramine is second-generation antihistamine. _____
2. First-generation antihistamines can cross the blood-brain barrier. _____
3. Blurry vision and dry eyes are anticholinergic side effects. _____
4. The -*atadine* stem indicates that a drug is an H_2 blocker. _____
5. Pseudoephedrine mimics the fight-or-flight system. _____
6. Oxymetazoline is an antihistamine for allergy. _____
7. Triamcinolone works in the same day, similar to oxymetazoline. _____
8. Guaifenesin is an antitussive to prevent cough. _____
9. Montelukast works as a leukotriene receptor blocker for chronic treatment of asthma. _____
10. The suffix -*mab* indicates a monoclonal antibody. _____

MULTIPLE CHOICE (10)

1. Which of these is a behind-the-counter item with daily and monthly limits on its purchase and relieves congestion quickly?
   a. loratadine (Claritin)
   b. pseudoephedrine (Sudafed)
   c. cetirizine (Zyrtec)
   d. phenylephrine (Sudafed PE)

2. Which medication is an over-the-counter (OTC) nasal steroid?
   a. guaifenesin (Mucinex)
   b. triamcinolone (Nasacort 24 HR)
   c. dextromethorphan (Delsym)
   d. oxymetazoline (Afrin)

3. Which medication affects leukotrienes for chronic asthma prophylaxis?
   a. fluticasone (Flovent HFA)
   b. montelukast (Singulair)
   c. albuterol (ProAir)
   d. tiotropium (Spiriva)

4. Which dosage form might be best for a small child who does not have the dexterity to actuate an MDI?
   a. dry powder inhaler
   b. respimat inhaler
   c. nebulizer
   d. metered-dose inhaler

5. Which asthma medicine contains a short-acting $beta_2$ agonist?
   a. albuterol (ProAir)
   b. tiotropium (Spiriva)
   c. fluticasone (Flovent HFA)
   d. fluticasone/salmeterol (Advair)

6. Which respiratory drug or drug combination contains a long-acting muscarinic antagonist?
   a. triamcinolone (Nasacort 24 HR)
   b. tiotropium (Spiriva)
   c. albuterol (ProAir)
   d. albuterol/ipratropium (DuoNeb)

7. All of these medicines block a histamine receptor. Which one is a very sedating, first-generation H_1 antihistamine?
   a. loratadine (Claritin)
   b. famotidine (Pepcid)
   c. montelukast (Singulair)
   d. diphenhydramine (Benadryl)

8. Which is a possible side effect of inhaled corticosteroids if the patient fails to rinse out their mouth after each use?
   a. dysphonia
   b. constipation
   c. gastroesophageal reflux disease
   d. diarrhea

9. Which medication contains a steroid?
   a. albuterol (ProAir)
   b. budesonide/formoterol (Symbicort)
   c. albuterol/ipratropium (DuoNeb)
   d. montelukast (Singulair)

10. We can expect _____ to last up to 24 hours.
    a. tiotropium (Spiriva)
    b. albuterol (ProAir)
    c. dextromethorphan (Delsym)
    d. guaifenesin (Mucinex)

MATCHING (5)

Match the chemical branches to the drug name.

1. _____ antihistamine, first-generation
2. _____ antihistamine, second-generation
3. _____ decongestant
4. _____ steroid
5. _____ leukotriene inhibitor

a. diphenhydramine
b. fluticasone
c. pseudoephedrine
d. loratadine
e. montelukast

COMPLETION (5)

1. Loratadine (Claritin) is an example of a(n) _____.

2. The steroid half of budesonide/formoterol is _____.

3. A long-acting anticholinergic is _____.

4. An anticholinergic effect includes _____.

5. Medications like _____ may help alleviate a cough.

a. budesonide
b. dry eyes
c. dextromethorphan
d. first-generation antihistamine
e. tiotropium

DOSAGE CALCULATIONS (5)

1. An adult is to take 20 mL every 4 hours of dextromethorphan. They have a 120-mL bottle. How long will the bottle last in hours?

2. A combination product has 200 mg of guaifenesin per dose and the patient is to take the medication no more than 12 times per day. What is the maximum dosage they would receive in a day of guaifenesin?

3. A older adult patient buys cetirizine (Zyrtec) liquid because they cannot swallow pills. The 120-mL bottle reads that they are to take 5 mL each day. How long will the bottle last?

4. A patient with chronic obstructive pulmonary disease is to take 500 mcg of ipratropium via nebulizer every 6 hours around the clock. If there are 500 mcg in 2.5 mL, how many mL of nebulizer solution will the patient use in a day?

5. There are 17 mcg of ipratropium in each actuation of the inhaler. If the patient is not to exceed 12 actuations per day, what is the total number of mcg the patient should not exceed in the day?

VISUAL CRITICAL THINKING (7)

1. Histamine – A Tale of 2 Receptors *(Place numbers 1 and 2 in the blanks as appropriate.)*

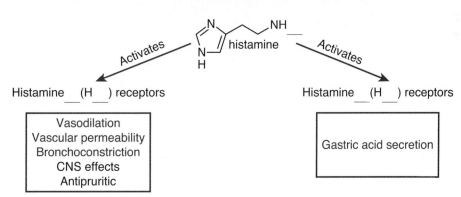

Histamine – A tale of 2 receptors

Biologically-active compound stored in mast cells and basophils released when allergen attaches to mast cells and basophils

Activates

histamine

Activates

Histamine ___ (H ___) receptors

Vasodilation
Vascular permeability
Bronchoconstriction
CNS effects
Antipruritic

Histamine ___ (H ___) receptors

Gastric acid secretion

2. Antihistamines – Types. Insert the terms *diphenhydramine, famotidine,* and *loratadine* in the figure.

Antihistamines – types

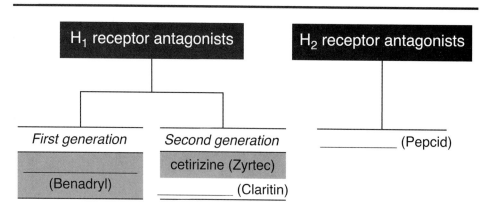

| H₁ receptor antagonists | | H₂ receptor antagonists |

First generation

_____

(Benadryl)

Second generation

cetirizine (Zyrtec)

_____ (Claritin)

_____ (Pepcid)

All antihistamines work best when started before symptoms appear

3. Expectorants – Guaifenesin. Insert the terms *codeine* and *dextromethorphan* in the figure.

Expectorants – guaifenesin

Guaifenesin

Increases the volume and decreases viscosity of respiratory mucus
- Makes it able to be coughed up easier
- Often added with antitussives

Combination antitussive & expectorant	
Over-the-counter	Prescription-only
guaifenesin/_____ (Robitussin DM)	guaifenesin/_____ (Cheratussin AC)

4. Asthma – Pathology. Insert the terms *allergen, bronchoconstriction,* and *inflammation* in the figure.

Asthma – Pathology

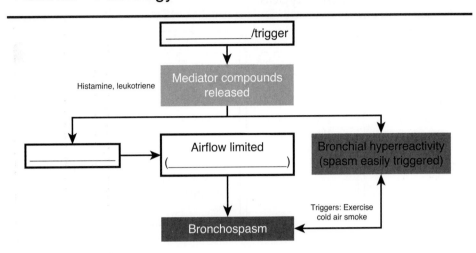

5. Asthma – Oral Glucocorticoids. Insert the terms *asthma* and *diabetic* in the figure. Terms may be used more than once.

Asthma – oral glucocorticoids

Oral steroids act through anti-inflammatory actions
Used for _____ exacerbations but not chronically, due to adverse effects

Prednisone

Short burst doses in _____
Available only as oral formulations

Methylprednisolone

Short burst doses
Available as:
- Oral tablet
- IV formulation

Notes:
Glucocorticoids can raise glucose levels, which must be watched closely by _____ patients

6. Asthma – Inhaler Types. Insert the terms *dexterity, dry powder, metered-dose, nebulizer, respimat,* and *yes* in the figure. Terms may be used more than once.

Asthma – inhaler types

_____ required: Moderate-high Propellant: _____	_____ required: Moderate Propellant: No, breath activated	Dexterity required: Low Propellant: No Unique: Mist created with pressure	Dexterity required: Minimal Propellant: No Unique: Mist created by stationary machine

7. Asthma – Combined Agents. Insert the terms *LABA* and *SABA* in the figure.

Asthma – combined agents

Combination inhalers allow for easier administration of medications
• Only have to use one product instead of each individually

ICS/_____   _____/SAMA

Fluticasone/salmeterol (Advair) Budesonide/formoterol (Symbicort)	Albuterol/ipratropium (DuoNeb)
[Inflammation/bronchoconstriction]	[Bronchoconstriction/bronchoconstriction]

Notes:
Patients using an inhaled corticosteroid (ICS) *must* rinse
their mouth after use!

MNEMONICS (1)

1. Name three decongestants including a decongestant/antihistamine combination. Outline the limit on days use for intranasal decongestants and a disease state to avoid with these medicines. Use the mnemonic STUFFED UP PEOPLE to help you remember.

STUFFED UP PEOPLE

P _____ (decongestant)

E _____ (days use limit)

O _____ (decongestant)

P _____ / (decongestant with)

L _____ (antihistamine)

E _____ U _____ H _____ (disease state to avoid)

11 Immune

TRUE FALSE (10)

1. Fluconazole is an azole antifungal. _____
2. A use for sulfamethoxazole and trimethoprim includes urinary tract infections. _____
3. We would avoid ciprofloxacin for infectious diarrhea. _____
4. The -floxacin stem indicates an antibiotic is a fluoroquinolone. _____
5. Linezolid interacts with SSRI antidepressants. _____
6. *Clostridium difficile* is a superinfection sometimes caused by clindamycin. _____
7. Doxycycline has the -*cycline* stem to identify it as a tetracycline. _____
8. Vancomycin is a penicillin antibiotic. _____
9. Ceftriaxone is a first-generation cephalosporin. _____
10. A narrow-spectrum antibiotic covers a wide range of organisms. _____

MULTIPLE CHOICE (10)

1. Which antibiotic drug class affects cell walls?
   a. fluoroquinolones
   b. penicillins
   c. macrolides
   d. aminoglycosides

2. A penicillin antibiotic with _____ can be effective against beta-lactamase bacterial enzymes.
   a. clavulanic acid
   b. hydrochloric acid
   c. tetracyclines
   d. macrolides

3. Which sulfonamide antibiotic would treat a simple urinary tract infection?
   a. linezolid (Zyvox)
   b. clindamycin (Cleocin)
   c. sulfamethoxazole/trimethoprim (Bactrim)
   d. ceftaroline (Teflaro)

4. Which medication is bactericidal?
   a. azithromycin (Z-Pak)
   b. amikacin (Amikin)
   c. minocycline (Minocin)
   d. linezolid (Zyvox)

5. Which is a tetracycline antibiotic?
   a. amikacin (Amikin)
   b. doxycycline (Doryx)
   c. linezolid (Zyvox)
   d. gentamicin (Garamycin)

6. Which atypical antibiotic will cause nausea and vomiting when mixed with alcohol?
   a. fluconazole (Diflucan)
   b. sulfamethoxazole/trimethoprim (Bactrim)
   c. metronidazole (Flagyl)
   d. amphotericin B (Fungizone)

7. Which azole antifungal is useful for vaginal yeast infections?
   a. amphotericin B (Fungizone)
   b. fluconazole (Diflucan)
   c. nystatin (Mycostatin)
   d. metronidazole (Flagyl)

8. Herpes simplex virus treatment involves which medication?
   a. palivizumab (Synagis)
   b. acyclovir (Zovirax)
   c. gentamicin (Garamycin)
   d. infliximab (Remicade)

9. What tuberculosis treatment will make the urine turn orange?
   a. rifampin
   b. isoniazid
   c. pyrazinamide
   d. ethambutol

10. In which class would azithromycin (Zithromax) fall?
    a. macrolide antibiotic
    b. azole antifungal
    c. integrase strand transfer inhibitor
    d. penicillin antibiotic

MATCHING (5)

Match the antibiotic to its drug class.

1. _____ amoxicillin
2. _____ doxycycline
3. _____ azithromycin
4. _____ sulfamethoxazole/trimethoprim
5. _____ gentamicin

a. sulfa drug
b. macrolide
c. tetracycline
d. aminoglycoside
e. penicillin

COMPLETION (5)

1. Amikacin (Amikin) is an example of a(n) _____.

2. The stem for an antiviral is _____.

3. The stem for a penicillin antibiotic is _____.

4. The stem for a cephalosporin antibiotic is _____.

5. A cell with a peptidoglycan layer is _____.

a. *-vir*
b. *cef-*
c. gram-negative
d. aminoglycoside
e. *-cillin*

DOSAGE CALCULATIONS (5)

1. The directions on an azithromycin pack, known as a Z-Pak, say that the patient is to take two 250-mg tablets on day one and one 250-mg tablet each day for 4 days thereafter. How many milligrams of medication will the patient take in total?

2. An infant Augmentin dose is 30 mg/kg/day divided every 12 hours. How many milligrams will be in each dose for a 4-kg infant?

3. A patient is to take 1 teaspoonful three times daily for 14 days. If each teaspoonful contains 5 mL, how many mL do they need to take in a day?

4. A patient is to get 2 mL of nystatin suspension four times a day. How many mL would they use in a week?

5. An amphotericin B dose is 0.3 mg/kg/dose IV daily to start. How many milligrams will there be in each dose for a 220-pound patient?

VISUAL CRITICAL THINKING (12)

1. Gram Positive vs Gram Negative. Place the terms *negative* and *positive* in the figure.

Gram Positive vs Gram Negative

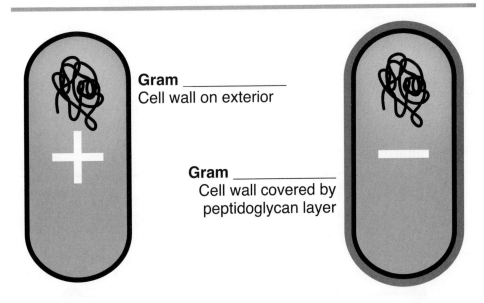

Gram _____
Cell wall on exterior

Gram _____
Cell wall covered by
peptidoglycan layer

2. Antimicrobials – Targets. Place the terms *bactericidal*, *bacteriostatic*, *cell wall*, and *DNA/RNA* in the figure.

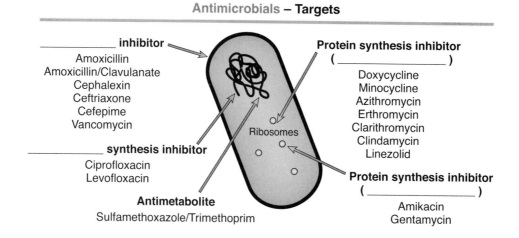

Antimicrobials – Targets

_____ inhibitor

Amoxicillin
Amoxicillin/Clavulanate
Cephalexin
Ceftriaxone
Cefepime
Vancomycin

_____ synthesis inhibitor

Ciprofloxacin
Levofloxacin

Antimetabolite
Sulfamethoxazole/Trimethoprim

Ribosomes

Protein synthesis inhibitor
(_____)

Doxycycline
Minocycline
Azithromycin
Erthromycin
Clarithromycin
Clindamycin
Linezolid

Protein synthesis inhibitor
(_____)
Amikacin
Gentamycin

3. Antimicrobial – Spectrums. Place the terms *broad* and *narrow* in the figure.

Antimicrobial – Spectrums

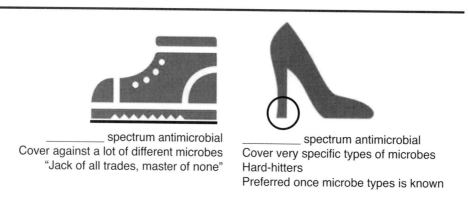

_____ spectrum antimicrobial
Cover against a lot of different microbes
"Jack of all trades, master of none"

_____ spectrum antimicrobial
Cover very specific types of microbes
Hard-hitters
Preferred once microbe types is known

4. Antibiotics – Cephalosporins. Place the terms *maxipime*, *rocephin*, and *teflaro* in the figure.

Antibiotics – cephalosporins

All have a β-lactam ring like penicillins
Work the same as penicillins-still inhibit cell wall synthesis

5 generations of cephalosporins

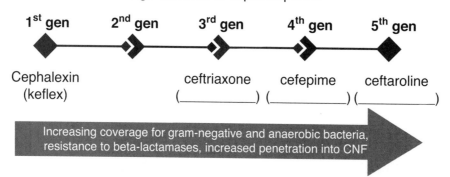

1st gen   2nd gen   3rd gen   4th gen   5th gen

Cephalexin   ceftriaxone   cefepime   ceftaroline
(keflex)   (_____)   (_____)   (_____)

Increasing coverage for gram-negative and anaerobic bacteria, resistance to beta-lactamases, increased penetration into CNF

5. Bacteriostatic vs. Bactericidal. Place the terms *bactericidal* and *bacteriostatic* in the figure.

Bacteriostatic vs bactericidal

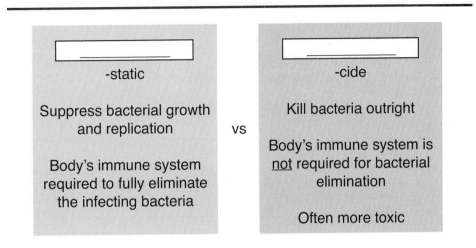

6. Bacteriostatic – Bacterial Ribosomes. Place the terms *30S* and *50S* in the figure.

Bacteriostatic – bacterial ribosomes

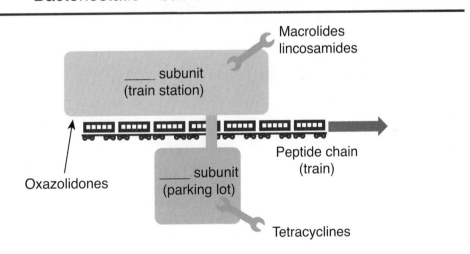

7. Antifungals – Overview. Place the terms *superficial* and *systemic* in the figure.

Antifungals – overview

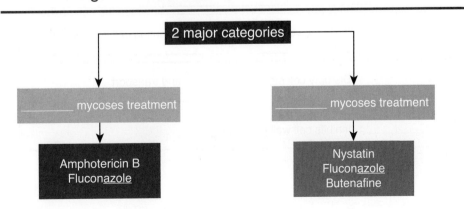

8. Antifungals – Azoles. Place the terms *azoles* and *polyenes* in the figure.

Antifungals – azoles

Fluconazole (diflucan)

Inhibits ergosterol synthesis, preventing cell membrane formation and causes increased membrane permeation

Used for both systemic and superficial fungal infections

<table>
<tr>
<td>_____
• Work on outside of membrane to bind to sterols and increase permeation
• Very toxic due to mammal sterol binding</td>
<td>_____
Work on inside of cell to prevent sterol formation and increase permeation
• Minimal toxicity due to only fungal uptake</td>
</tr>
</table>

9. Tuberculosis – Pathology. Place the terms *active* and *latent* in the figure.

Tuberculosis – **Pathology**

Bacteria covered in a waxy, mycolic acid shell (giving them the name *myco*bacteria)
Require oxygen-rich environments, making them respiratory infectors
Both versions of TB must be treated:

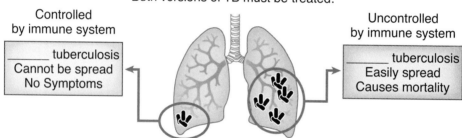

Controlled by immune system

_____ tuberculosis
Cannot be spread
No Symptoms

Uncontrolled by immune system

_____ tuberculosis
Easily spread
Causes mortality

10. Antimycobacterial Agents. Place the terms *ethambutol, isoniazid, pyrazinamide,* and *rifampin* in the figure.

Antimycobacterial agents

_____: Prevents RNA synthesis Causes harmless, orange-red coloration to bodily fluids
_____: Inhibits mycolic acid synthesis, preventing cell wall formation
_____: Disrupts cell membrane function and transport
_____: Inhibits cell wall formation

11. Antivirals – Targets. Place the terms *attachment, release,* and *synthesis* in the figure.

Antivirals – **Targets**

Viruses are obligate parasites, making them challenging to treat
  • Rely entirely upon host cells and synthetic commands
    for replication

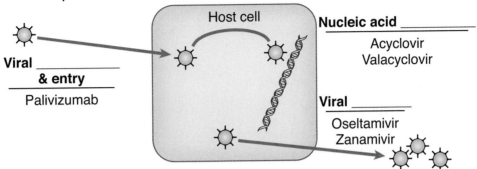

Viral _____
_____ **& entry**
Palivizumab

Host cell

Nucleic acid _____
Acyclovir
Valacyclovir

Viral _____
Oseltamivir
Zanamivir

12. Antivirals – HIV Replication Cycle. Place the terms *attachment, budding, fusion,* and *processing* in the figure.

Antivirals – HIV replication cycle

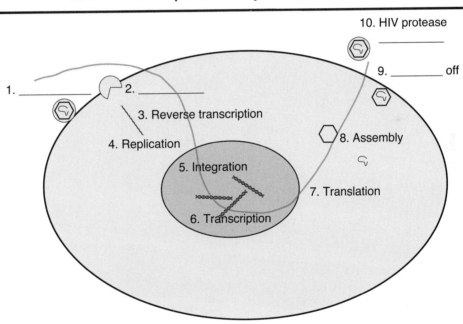

10. HIV protease
_____

9. _____ off

1. _____

2. _____

3. Reverse transcription

4. Replication

8. Assembly

5. Integration

7. Translation

6. Transcription

1. Name seven HIV medications in order of attack to the host cell. Use the mnemonic THEM THREE RAID HIV to help you remember.

THEM THREE, RAID HIV

T _____ and quad therapy

H

E _____ (Fusion inhibitor)

M _____ (CCR5 receptor antagonist)

T _____ (NRTI)

H

R

E _____ (NNRTI)

E _____ (NNRTI)

Ra _____ (Integrase inhibitor)

I

D _____ (Protease inhibitor)

HIV

12 Neuropsychology

TRUE FALSE (10)

1. An SSRI affects both serotonin and norepinephrine. _____
2. Atomoxetine is an MAO inhibitor. _____
3. Bupropion is for depression and smoking cessation. _____
4. Clonazepam is an antidepressant. _____
5. Dexmethylphenidate has an indication for attention-deficit/hyperactivity disorder (ADHD). _____
6. Eszopiclone is a treatment for insomnia. _____
7. Lithium is for depression. _____
8. Ramelteon has no effect on melatonin. _____
9. Varenicline has no side effects with its use. _____
10. We expect that an amide would be more allergenic than an ester local anesthetic. _____

MULTIPLE CHOICE (10)

1. A medication that ends in -*oxetine* could be a(n): *(Select all that apply.)*
   a. local anesthetic.
   b. SSRI.
   c. SNRI.
   d. lenzodiazepine.

2. If a prescriber is going to provide a benzodiazepine for their patient, which is correct?
   a. clonazepam
   b. ramelteon
   c. paroxetine
   d. diphenhydramine

3. It would be appropriate for a patient to use which medication in the evening?
   a. caffeine
   b. methylphenidate
   c. dexmethylphenidate
   d. eszopiclone

4. An antidepressant that affects two neurotransmitters is:
   a. escitalopram.
   b. venlafaxine.
   c. citalopram.
   d. paroxetine.

5. An antidepressant that also helps patients quit smoking is:
   a. lorazepam.
   b. bupropion.
   c. varenicline.
   d. citalopram.

6. The best medication for a patient with ADHD would be:
   a. citalopram.
   b. paroxetine.
   c. fluoxetine.
   d. atomoxetine.

7. Which represents a stimulant medication for ADHD?
   a. alprazolam
   b. atomoxetine
   c. dexmethylphenidate
   d. clonazepam

8. Which represents a sedative-hypnotic?
   a. paroxetine
   b. zolpidem
   c. escitalopram
   d. alprazolam

9. Nystagmus and gingival hyperplasia are both concerns with which medication?
   a. divalproex
   b. lithium
   c. phenytoin
   d. carbamazepine

10. A medicine that is a precursor to dopamine is:
    a. citalopram.
    b. carbidopa.
    c. selegiline.
    d. levodopa.

MATCHING (5)

Match the antidepressant to its drug class.

1. _____ amitriptyline
2. _____ bupropion
3. _____ isocarboxazid
4. _____ paroxetine
5. _____ venlafaxine

a. atypical
b. MAOI
c. SNRI
d. TCA
e. SSRI

COMPLETION (5)

1. An antidepressant named after a shape is _____.

2. Escitalopram (Lexapro) is an example of a(n) _____.

3. The stem for amitriptyline is _____.

4. The stem for paroxetine is _____.

5. The stem for venlafaxine is _____.

a. *-faxine*
b. *-triptyline*
c. TCA
d. SSRI
e. *-oxetine*

DOSAGE CALCULATIONS (5)

1. A patient needs to take fluoxetine 20 mg daily for 30 days and it comes as a 20 mg/5 mL liquid. How many mL should the patient have to ensure they have enough medicine for 30 days?

2. A maximum dose of levodopa is 8000 mg/day. If a patient has 250-mg tablets, how many would they need to take to reach the 8000 mg?

3. A patient is switching from citalopram to escitalopram and needs half the dose. Currently, the patient has 40 mg of citalopram once daily. How much citalopram will they need as a daily dose?

4. A patient is given alprazolam 0.5 mg, to be taken as needed. If the patient needs to use the medication no more than 14 days per month, how many milligrams do they need to make sure they have enough?

5. A patient takes lithium 400 mg twice daily with food. The prescription is changed to 400 mg three times daily. How many milligrams does the patient now take in a day?

VISUAL CRITICAL THINKING (11)

1. Neuro/Psych – Medication Targets. Place the terms *axonal* and *synaptic* in the figure.

Neuro/Psych – Medication Targets

The two different steps to neuron signal transmission are the largets for medications

_____ Conduction	_____ Trasmission
Drugs are not selective (all axons work basically the same)	Can be very selective, working on different synapses and specific neurotransmitters
• Lots of adverse effects	Most metications work on this target
Very few medications inhibit this transmission	

2. Neuro/Psych – Local Anesthetics. Place the terms *amide* and *ester* in the figure.

Neuro/Psych – local anesthetics

Two common local anesthetics

Non-selective axonal conduction inhibitors - stop the action potential and block neurotransmitter release

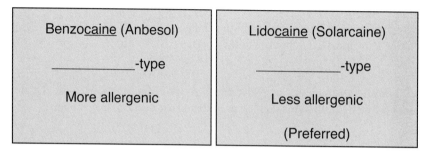

Benzocaine (Anbesol)	Lidocaine (Solarcaine)
_____ -type	_____ -type
More allergenic	Less allergenic
	(Preferred)

3. Sedative-Hypnotics – Overview. Place the terms *hypnotic* and *sedative* in the figure below.

Sedative-hypnotics – overview

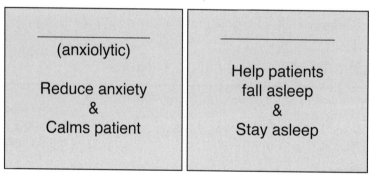

_____ (anxiolytic)	_____
Reduce anxiety & Calms patient	Help patients fall asleep & Stay asleep

Some medications are sedative or hypnotic, others are both

4. Neuro/Psych – Antidepressants. Place the terms *MAOIs, SNRIs, SSRIs,* and *TCAs* in the figure.

Neuro/Psych – antidepressants

All antidepressants work to increase levels of monoamines lowered in depression

Selective serotonin reuptake inhibitors (_____)	Serotonin-norepinephrine reuptake inhibitors (_____)
Four antidepressant classes (excluding atypical)	
Tricyclic antidepressants (_____)	Monoamine oxidase inhibitors (_____)

5. Serotonergic Agents Timing. Place the terms *escitalopram*, *paroxetine*, and *sertraline* in the figure.

Serotonergic agents timing

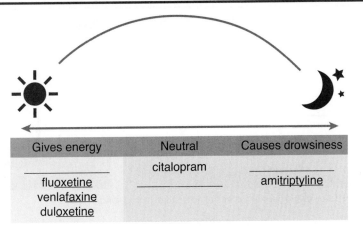

Gives energy	Neutral	Causes drowsiness
_____	citalopram	_____
fluoxetine	_____	amitriptyline
venlafaxine		
duloxetine		

isocarboxazid given twice daily

6. ADHD – Overview. Place the terms *ADHD* and *Non-ADHD* in the figure.

ADHD – Overview

Attention Deficit Hyperactive Disorder (ADHD)

Prefrontal Cortex
• Planning
• Problem solving
• Short-term memory
• Behavior

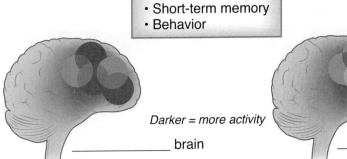

Darker = more activity

_____ brain   _____ brain

7. Neuro/Psych – Antipsychotics. Place the terms *1st generation* and *2nd generation* in the figure.

Neuro/psych – Antipsychotics

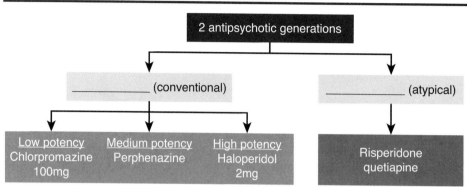

Potency – required dose, low potency is not less effective than high potency!

8. Neuro/Psych – 1st Gen Antipsychotics. Place the terms *high* and *low* in the figure.

Neuro/Psych – 1st gen antipsychotics

Can block CNS acetylcholine, dopamine, histamine, and norepinephrine. Blocking dopamine can lead to extrapyramidal effects (EPS) which can be permanent. **EPS examples include:**

1. Acute dystonia – day + tonia = bad + muscles (spasms back, face, neck, tongue)
2. Parkinsonism – looks like parkinson's disease, but shares symptoms
3. Akathisia – literally "dance" = restlessness. NOT akinesia, lack of movement
4. Tardive dyskinesia – late + bad + movement = choreoatheiod movements

Drug name	Potency	Sedation	*EPS potential*
chlorpromazine (Thorazine)	_____	_____	*Moderate*
haloperidol (Haldol)	_____	_____	*Very high*

9. Epilepsy – Carbamazepine. Place the terms *grapefruit, marrow,* and *teratogenic* in the figure.

Epilepsy – **Carbamazepine**

Carbamazepine (Tegretol)

• Inhibits sodium channels on hyperactive neurons
  • Prevents sodium from entering neuron, stopping action potential
• Serious drug reactions:

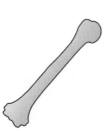
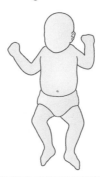
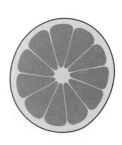

| Bone _____ suppression | _____ | _____ juice increases levels |

10. Parkinson's Disease – Presentation. Place the terms *bradykinesis, postural,* and *rigidity* in the figure.

Parkinson's Disease – **Presentation**

Low dopamine/high acetylcholine result in:

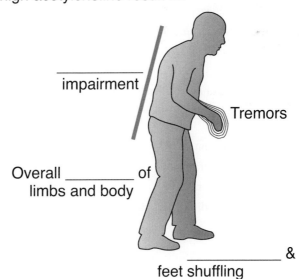

_____ impairment

Tremors

Overall _____ of limbs and body

_____ & feet shuffling

11. AD – Pathology. Place the terms *acetylcholine, beta amyloid plaques,* and *microtubules* in the figure.

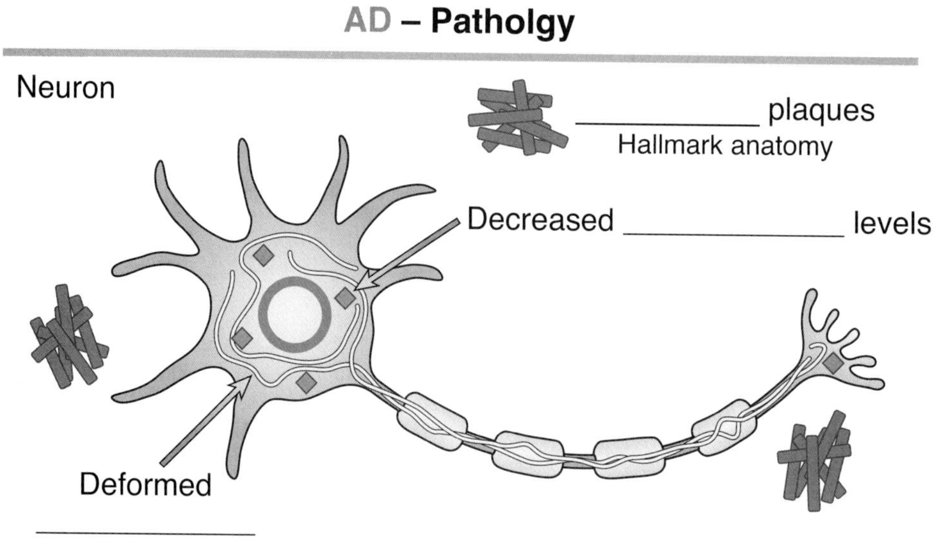

AD – Patholgy

Neuron

_____ plaques
Hallmark anatomy

Decreased _____ levels

Deformed

_____

MNEMONICS (2)

1. Name four benzodiazepine anxiolytics. Use the mnemonic BE CALM to help you remember.

BE CALM

Buspirone (nonbenzodiazepine)

Extended time to work (concern)

C_____ (benzodiazepine)

A_____ (benzodiazepine)

L_____ (benzodiazepine)

M_____ (benzodiazepine)

2. Name two medications for smoking cessation and a single side effect or drug–disease interaction for both. Use the mnemonic STOP SMOKING VIBE to help you remember.

STOP SMOKING VIBE

V_____ (medication)

I _____ (side effect)

B_____ (medication)

E _____ (drug–disease interaction)

13 Cardiology

TRUE FALSE (10)

1. All warfarin tablets come in the same peach color. _____
2. Alpha blockers have effectiveness in benign prostatic hyperplasia and hypertension. _____
3. Antihyperlipidemics include nifedipine and amlodipine. _____
4. Clopidogrel uses the *clop-* prefix to indicate it works as an antiplatelet agent. _____
5. Furosemide works at the ascending loop of Henle. _____
6. Mannitol is an example of a loop diuretic. _____
7. Potassium-sparing diuretics would include spironolactone. _____
8. Side effects of nondihydropyridines include constipation and bradycardia. _____
9. The renin-angiotensin-aldosterone system (RAAS) maintains fluid and salt levels in the body. _____
10. The stem for an angiotensin-converting enzyme (ACE) inhibitor is *-olol*. _____

MULTIPLE CHOICE (10)

1. Which medication is a thiazide diuretic?
   a. furosemide (Lasix)
   b. amlodipine (Norvasc)
   c. spironolactone (Aldactone)
   d. hydrochlorothiazide (Microzide)

2. Which diuretic preserves potassium levels?
   a. furosemide (Lasix)
   b. spironolactone (Aldactone)
   c. hydrochlorothiazide (Microzide)
   d. triamterene (Dyrenium)

3. What stem would you expect for an ACE inhibitor?
   a. *-dipine*
   b. *-pril*
   c. *-sartan*
   d. *-olol*

4. Which medication is a nondihydropyridine calcium channel blocker (CCB)?
   a. furosemide (Lasix)
   b. nifedipine (Procardia)
   c. verapamil (Calan)
   d. amlodipine (Norvasc)

5. Fill in the blanks with the correct words: _____ affect the vessels and heart, while _____ affect the vessels only.
   a. Dihydropyridines; dihydropyridines
   b. Nondihydropyridines; dihydropyridines
   c. Nondihydropyridines; nondihydropyridines
   d. Dihydropyridines; nondihydropyridines

6. Which medication is a first-generation beta blocker?
   a. carvedilol
   b. metoprolol tartrate
   c. metoprolol succinate
   d. propranolol

7. Fill in the correct words for the following blanks: Anticoagulants affect coagulation in the moving _____ vessels, while antiplatelets affect the _____.
   a. slower, arteries
   b. faster, arteries
   c. slower, veins
   d. faster, veins

8. Which is a parenteral anticoagulant?
   a. heparin
   b. dabigatran
   c. clopidogrel
   d. warfarin

9. Which antiplatelet is found over the counter?
   a. warfarin
   b. enoxaparin
   c. clopidogrel
   d. aspirin

10. Blocking which receptor might reduce blood pressure?
    a. alpha
    b. gamma
    c. delta
    d. epsilon

MATCHING (5)

Match the antihypertensive to its drug class.

1. _____ carvedilol
2. _____ diltiazem
3. _____ furosemide
4. _____ nifedipine
5. _____ propranolol

a. nondihydropyridine CCB
b. dihydropyridine CCB
c. third-generation beta blocker
d. loop diuretic
e. first-generation beta blocker

COMPLETION (5)

1. A CCB that affects the heart and vessels _____.

2. A CCB that only affects the vessels is _____.

3. A diuretic that works at the ascending loop of Henle is _____.

4. A diuretic that works at the distal convoluted tubule is _____.

5. An ACE inhibitor is _____.

a. lisinopril
b. diltiazem
c. furosemide
d. HCTZ
e. nifedipine

DOSAGE CALCULATIONS (5)

1. If a patient has a heparin drip running at 25 mL/hour and the 250-mL bag has 25,000 units of heparin, how many hourly units is the patient receiving?

2. A heparin bag has 25,000 units in 500 mL. The patient needs 1500 units hourly. How many mL per hour should the patient receive?

3. A patient needs 7.5 mg of warfarin on Monday, Wednesday, and Thursday, and 5 mg on every other day. How many 5-mg tablets does the patient need for a 28-day supply?

4. A patient needs to take 40 mg twice daily of furosemide. How many tablets does the patient need for a 30-day supply of 20-mg tablets?

5. Over 4 weeks, a patient will increase their nifedipine dose from 30 mg to 120 mg increasing the dose by 30 mg each week. How many 30-mg tablets does the patient need to complete this regimen?

VISUAL CRITICAL THINKING (9)

1. Cardiovascular System – Overview. Place the terms *arteries, capillaries,* and *veins* in the figure.

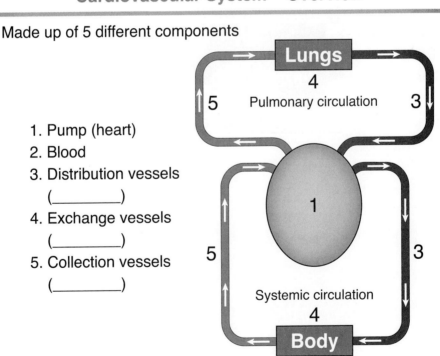

Cardiovascular System – Overview

Made up of 5 different components

1. Pump (heart)
2. Blood
3. Distribution vessels
   (_____)
4. Exchange vessels
   (_____)
5. Collection vessels
   (_____)

Lungs
4
Pulmonary circulation

Systemic circulation
4
Body

2. Cardiovascular System – Cardiac Output. Place the terms *output, rate,* and *volume* in the figure.

Cardiovascular System – **Cardiac Output**

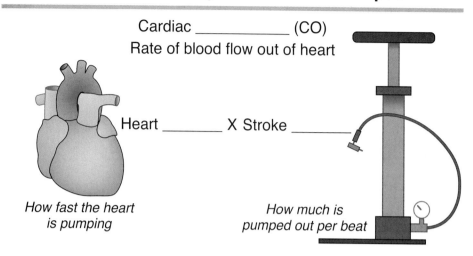

Cardiac _____ (CO)
Rate of blood flow out of heart

Heart _____ X Stroke _____

*How fast the heart
is pumping*

*How much is
pumped out per beat*

3. Cardiovascular System – Pressure. Place the terms *diastolic* and *systolic* in the figure.

Cardiovascular System – **Pressure**

Arterial Pressure (Blood Pressure)
Pressure of the blood on the arterial walls

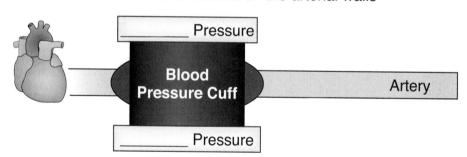

_____ Pressure

**Blood
Pressure Cuff**

Artery

_____ Pressure

4. Kidneys – Diuretic Sites of Action. Place the terms *furosemide, HCTZ, mannitol,* and *spironolactone* in the figure.

Kidneys – Diuretic Sites of Action

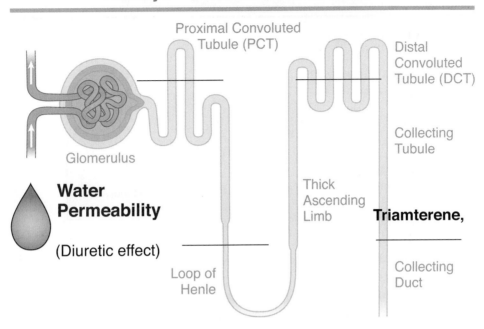

Water Permeability

(Diuretic effect)

Glomerulus

Proximal Convoluted Tubule (PCT)

Distal Convoluted Tubule (DCT)

Collecting Tubule

Thick Ascending Limb

Triamterene,

Loop of Henle

Collecting Duct

5. RAAS – Overview. Place the terms *ACE* and *ARB* in the figure. Terms may be used more than once.

RAAS – Overview

Low arterial pressure
Low sodium

Angiotensinogen | Renin | Angiotensin I

Inhibitors
Angiotensin Converting Enzyme

Angiotensin II

Na, H$_2$O reabsorption

Angiotensin receptor Blockers (_____)

Construction

Angiotensin receptor Blockers (_____)

Arteries

6. Hypertension – β-receptor antagonists. Place the terms *bronchial smooth muscle* and *heart* in the figure.

Hypertension – β-receptor antagonists

AKA the β-blockers

2 different β receptors: β_1 and β_2

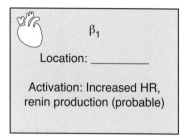
β_1

Location: _____

Activation: Increased HR, renin production (probable)

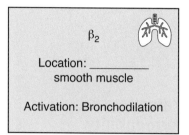
β_2

Location: _____
smooth muscle

Activation: Bronchodilation

7. Hypertension – β-receptor antagonists. Place the terms *atenolol, carvedilol,* and *propranolol* in the figure.

Hypertension – β-receptor antagonists

1st generation	2nd generation	3rd generation
_____ (Inderal)	_____ (Tenormin) metoprolol tartrate (Lopressor) metoprolol succinate (Toprol XL)	_____ (Coreg)
Non-selective β_1 and β_2 blocker	Selective β_1 blockers	Selective β_1 blocker AND α_1-blockage

Most common adverse drug reaction for all generations: bradycardia

8. Coagulation Cascade – Overview. Place the terms *extrinsic* and *intrinsic* in the figure.

Coagulation cascade – Overview

Interaction between different proteins (factors) to cause fibrin to be deposited at tissue injury site

Proteins were named as roman numerals (Factor VI, etc) and were numbered based on discovery, not function
• *Cascade does not follow numerical order*

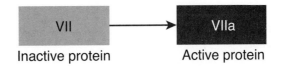

VII
Inactive protein

VIIa
Active protein

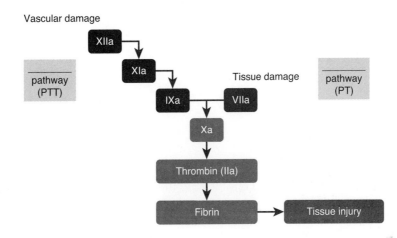

Vascular damage

XIIa

_____ pathway (PTT)

XIa

IXa

Tissue damage

VIIa

_____ pathway (PT)

Xa

Thrombin (IIa)

Fibrin → Tissue injury

9. Coagulation Cascade – *continued*. Place the terms *dabigatran, heparin,* and *warfarin* in the figure.

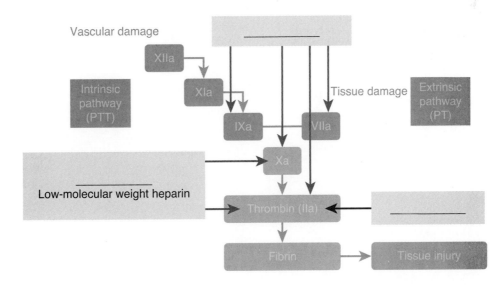

Vascular damage

XIIa

Intrinsic pathway (PTT)

XIa

IXa

Tissue damage

VIIa

Extrinsic pathway (PT)

Xa

Low-molecular weight heparin

Thrombin (IIa)

Fibrin → Tissue injury

1. Name six drug classes we can use to treat hypertension. Use the mnemonic ABCD to help you remember.

ABCD

A_____, (RAAS drug acronym)

A_____, (RAAS drug acronym) and

A_____ B_____ (adrenergic antagonist)

B_____ B_____ (adrenergic antagonist)

C_____ C_____ B_____

D_____

2. Name two potential side effects of HMG Co-As and whether you should use them in pregnancy. Use the mnemonic HMG Co-A to help you remember.

HMG Co-A

H_____ (side effect)

M_____ and rhabdomyolysis (side effect)

G_____, don't use in pregnancy

Cholesterol LDL lowering therapeutic effect

Onset of depression is controversial

Affects the enzyme HMG Co-A

14 Endocrine

TRUE FALSE (10)

1. Hypoglycemia is a condition of too much blood sugar. _____
2. One way medications target organs in diabetes is stopping liver glucose production. _____
3. Metformin is not associated with GI effects. _____
4. The islets of Langerhans are in the small intestine. _____
5. Glucagon helps when the blood sugar is dangerously low. _____
6. Regular insulin and rapid-acting insulin are the same. _____
7. Propylthiouracil is effective in reducing thyroid hormone. _____
8. Testosterone side effects include acne breakout, enlarged prostate, and possible gynecomastia. _____
9. Antimuscarinics for overactive bladder (OAB) include oxybutynin and tolterodine. _____
10. Dutasteride and finasteride are for erectile dysfunction (ED). _____

MULTIPLE CHOICE (10)

1. Which antidiabetic medicine is most likely to cause gastrointestinal distress?
   a. glyburide (DiaBeta)
   b. insulin glargine (Lantus)
   c. metformin (Glucophage)
   d. NPH insulin (Humulin N)

2. Although this insulin is in the pharmacy refrigerator, it is an over-the-counter (OTC) product.
   a. regular Insulin (Humulin R)
   b. insulin lispro (Humalog)
   c. insulin glargine (Lantus)
   d. glucagon (GlucaGen)

3. Which insulin is long-acting?
   a. regular insulin (Humulin R)
   b. insulin lispro (Humalog)
   c. NPH insulin (Humulin N)
   d. insulin glargine (Lantus)

4. A medication for hyperthyroidism is _____, while a medication for hypothyroidism is _____.
   a. insulin glargine (Lantus), metformin (Glucophage)
   b. metformin (Glucophage, insulin glargine (Lantus)
   c. levothyroxine (Synthroid), propylthiouracil (PTU)
   d. propylthiouracil (PTU), levothyroxine (Synthroid)

5. Which additional instructions would you give a patient who was recently started on a combination oral contraceptive (OC)?
   a. "Take this medication with food."
   b. "Cover the application area to avoid transfer to children."
   c. "This medication contains estrogen and progestin."
   d. "This is an oral medication that should be taken with water."

6. Which birth control medication is an example of emergency contraception?
   a. etonogestrel/ethinyl estradiol (NuvaRing)
   b. levonorgestrel (Mirena)
   c. norelgestromin/ethinyl estradiol (Xulane)
   d. levonorgestrel (Plan B One-Step)

7. One would expect an anticholinergic like oxybutynin (Ditropan) to cause _____.
   a. hypersalivation
   b. diarrhea
   c. lacrimation
   d. urinary retention

8. Which medication for OAB might cause dry eyes, constipation, and dry mouth?
   a. sildenafil (Viagra)
   b. tolterodine (Detrol)
   c. finasteride (Proscar)
   d. tamsulosin (Flomax)

9. Which medication acts as an alpha blocker?
   a. solifenacin (VESIcare)
   b. finasteride (Proscar)
   c. tamsulosin (Flomax)
   d. sildenafil (Viagra)

10. A dangerous interaction exists between nitroglycerin and which class of ED medications?
    a. losartan, an angiotensin receptor blocker (ARB)
    b. enalapril, an angiotensin-converting enzyme inhibitor (ACEI)
    c. nifedipine, a calcium channel blocker
    d. PDE5 inhibitor

MATCHING (5)

Match the medication to the disease state it treats.

1. _____ Glucagon
2. _____ Glucophage
3. _____ levothyroxine
4. _____ propylthiouracil
5. _____ sildenafil

a. hyperthyroidism
b. hypothyroidism
c. hyperglycemia
d. hypoglycemia
e. ED

COMPLETION (5)

1. An antidiabetic that reduces blood sugar is _____.

2. A medication that helps with benign prostatic hyperplasia (BPH) is _____.

3. A thyroid replacement hormone is _____.

4. A phosphodiesterase-5 (PDE-5) inhibitor is _____.

5. An insulin type is_____.

a. glargine
b. metformin
c. levothyroxine
d. sildenafil
e. alfuzosin

DOSAGE CALCULATIONS (5)

1. A patient needs to cover their carbohydrate (CHO) at a meal where their CHO insulin dose = the CHO grams in a meal / grams of CHO that 1 unit of insulin disposes. If the total carbohydrate grams in the meal is 70 and the grams of CHO disposed by 1 unit of insulin is 10, what is the CHO insulin dose?

2. If one unit of insulin will drop the blood sugar by 50 mg/dL (points) and the current blood sugar is 270 mg/dL, but the target is 120 mg/dL, then how many units will the patient need to reduce their blood sugar to the target?

3. What is the total insulin dose at a meal if one must add a CHO insulin dose of 4 units and a high blood sugar correction dose of 2 units?

4. One way to calculate the daily insulin requirement is to divide a patient's body weight in pounds by 4. If a patient weighs 196 pounds, what is their insulin requirement?

5. Another way to calculate the daily insulin requirement is to use 0.55 x the patient's weight in kilograms. What would the dose be for a patient who weighs 89 kilograms?

   Bonus: Compare the results from question numbers 4 and 5. Using the conversion of 2.2 pounds per kilogram, how many kilograms is a 196-pound patient?

VISUAL CRITICAL THINKING (9)

1. Diabetes mellitus (DM) – Pathology. Place the terms *gestational, type I,* and *type II* in the figure.

Diabetes mellitus (DM) – pathology

_____	_____	_____
Pancreas doesn't produce insulin	Insulin is produced but not utilized efficiently	Insulin is produced but not utilized efficiently
Usually diagnosed in childhood	Traditionally diagnosed in adulthood – seeing in children now	Occurs during pregnancy & continues shortly after delivery
Treatment **requires** insulin	Treatment starts with oral medications	Treated like type II

2. DM – Pathology. Place the terms *insulin, intestinal, liver, pancreatic,* and *sensitivity* in the figure.

DM – **Pathology**

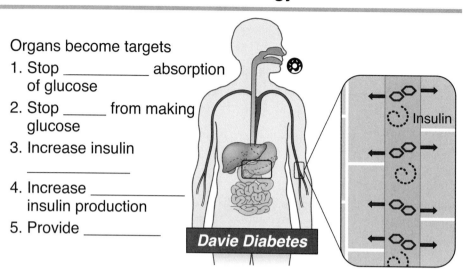

Organs become targets
1. Stop _____ absorption of glucose
2. Stop _____ from making glucose
3. Increase insulin _____
4. Increase _____ insulin production
5. Provide _____

Davie Diabetes

Insulin

3. Insulin – Comparison. Place the terms *glargine, lispro, NPH,* and *regular* in the figure.

Insulin – comparison

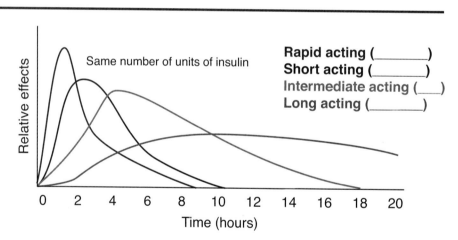

Same number of units of insulin

Rapid acting (_____)
Short acting (_____)
Intermediate acting (___)
Long acting (_____)

4. Thyroid Disorders – Pathology. Place the terms *high* and *low* in the figure.

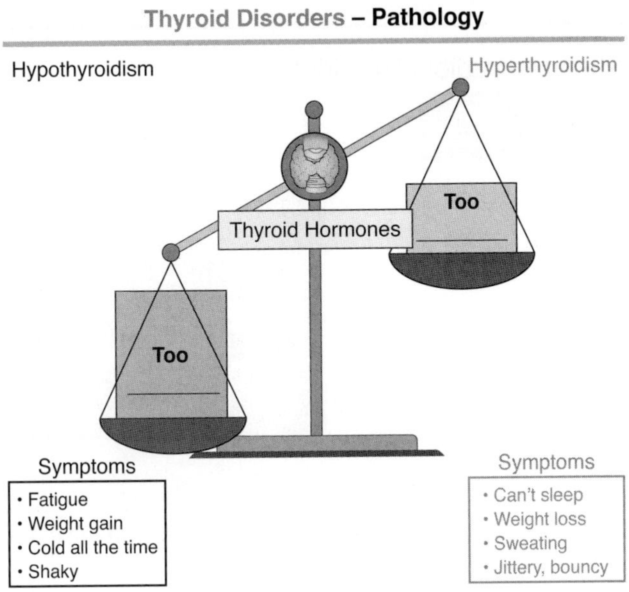

Thyroid Disorders – Pathology

Hypothyroidism

Hyperthyroidism

Thyroid Hormones

Too
_____

Too
_____

Symptoms
- Fatigue
- Weight gain
- Cold all the time
- Shaky

Symptoms
- Can't sleep
- Weight loss
- Sweating
- Jittery, bouncy

5. Hormonal Contraceptives – Combined. Place the terms *estrogen, iron,* and *progestin* in the figure.

Hormonal contraceptives – combined

Norethindrone/ethinyl estradiol/ferrous fumarate (Loestrin 24 FE)

_____
Norethindrone

_____
Ethinyl estradiol

_____
replacement

Same hormone amounts in
active pills for 24 of 28 days of
cycle to reduce length of
menstruation

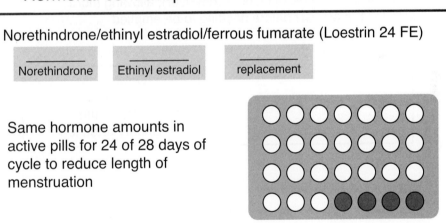

6. Hormonal Contraceptives – Combined. Place the terms *beginning* and *end* in the figure.

Hormonal contraceptives – combined

Norgestimate/ethinyl estradiol (Tri-sprintec)

Three different hormone amounts over 21 days, each 7 days long
• More estrogen at _____
• More progestin at _____
• Last week is placebo
Why do this?

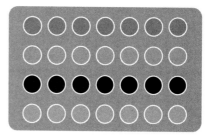

7. OAB – Antimuscarinics. Place the terms *oxybutynin, solifenacin,* and *tolterodine* in the figure.

OAB – antimuscarinics

_____ (Oxytrol, Ditropan)
_____ (Vesicare)
_____ (Detrol)

Relax smooth muscle of bladder (detrusor), allowing more urine to fill in bladder before needing to be emptied

Indications	Adverse drug reactions
Overactive bladder	Drowsiness Confusion Dry mouth Urinary retention

8. BPH – 5-Alpha Reductase Inhibitors. Place the terms *dutasteride* and *finasteride* in the figure.

BPH – 5-alpha reductase inhibitors

_____ (Avodart)
_____ (Proscar)

Decrease hormone production the prostate uses to grow
• Eventually leads to prostate shrinkage

Indications	Adverse drug reactions
Benign prostate hyperplasia	Decreased libido Erectile dysfunction

9. ED – Phosphodiesterase-5 (PDE-5) Inhibitors. Place the terms *sildenafil* and *tadalafil* in the figure.

ED – phosphodiesterase-5 (PDE-5) inhibitors

_____ (Viagra) – taken 1 hour before needed
_____ (Cialis) – taken 1 hours before needed, lasts 72 hours

Increase penile blood flow through nitric oxide-induced vasodilation

Indications	Adverse drug reactions
Erectile dysfunction	Headache Flushing Hypotension

1. Write a stem for an estrogen, a progestin, and a steroid. Name four birth control products: one that adds iron, one that is triphasic, one that uses a ring, and a fourth that is a patch. Name the active ingredient in a "morning-after pill." Name a steroid that has a gel vehicle for delivery. Use the mnemonic ESTER JUST STARES to help you remember.

Hormones and birth control

1. Estrogen stem - _____

2. Progestin stem - _____

3. Steroid stem - _____

Birth control products

1. _____ - adds iron

2. _____ - triphasic

3. _____ - uses a ring

4. _____ - is a patch

Active ingredient in "morning-after pill"

_____

Steroid with gel vehicle for delivery

_____

15 Pediatric Pharmacology

TRUE FALSE (20)

1. It is essential to consult a doctor if an infant younger than 3 months has a fever. _____
2. One resource used for treating pediatric diseases is *Pediatric Drug Formulations*. _____
3. Pediatric dosing is always based on age. _____
4. Dosing for pediatric patient A is the same as dosing for pediatric patient B. _____
5. Amoxicillin is often used to treat pharyngitis. _____
6. Even if dosing exceeds the maximum daily dose, it is appropriate to give to a pediatric patient. _____
7. A standard pharmacologic treatment of fever is acetaminophen. _____
8. For acute otitis media, only fever-reducing medications are used. _____
9. A typical vaccine a patient receives in early childhood is DTaP. _____
10. Group B strep can be treated with acetaminophen. _____
11. Acetaminophen's weight-based dosing is 10 to 15 mg/kg/dose every 4-6 hours. _____
12. Another term for a middle ear infection is otitis media. _____
13. Clark's Rule involves using an adult dose and a child's age. _____
14. Converting from pounds to kilograms requires a conversion of 2.2 kilograms per pound. _____
15. Most parents can accurately describe a child's weight. _____
16. The average body temperature is 37° Celsius. _____
17. Pharyngitis is another term for sore throat. _____
18. There is significant data published on pediatric medications regarding appropriate dosing. _____
19. When taking the temperature of an infant 3 months old or younger, the parent should measure it rectally. _____
20. Young's Rule requires using a child's weight and an adult dose. _____

MULTIPLE CHOICE (20)

1. For pediatric patients, which measure is used to ensure the drug dosage is safe and effective?
   a. body mass index
   b. blood pressure
   c. weight
   d. height

2. Which are resources used to treat pediatric diseases? *(Select all that apply.)*
   a. *Pediatric Dosage Handbook*
   b. *Allen's Compounded Formulations*
   c. *Clark's Compounded Formulations*
   d. *Children's Hospital of Philadelphia: Extemporaneous Formulations for Oral Administration*

3. _____-based dosing is commonly used for dosing pediatric patients, where conversions are used such as each _____ equals _____.
   a. Height; inch; 2.54 centimeters
   b. Weight; kilogram; 2.2 pounds
   c. Age; year; 365 days
   d. Body surface area; kilogram; 1 meter squared

4. Which formula(s) are used for pediatric dosing? *(Select all that apply.)*
   a. Young's Rule
   b. Smith's Rule
   c. Clark's Rule
   d. Ford's Rule

5. A patient diagnosed with a middle ear infection with a penicillin allergy can be given: *(Select all that apply.)*
   a. amoxicillin.
   b. amoxicillin-clavulanate.
   c. azithromycin.
   d. clindamycin.

6. To minimize dosing errors, pharmacists often provide: *(Select all that apply.)*
   a. household measures.
   b. marked syringes.
   c. household teaspoons.
   d. counseling.

7. Which causes a sore throat?
   a. group A beta-hemolytic streptococcus
   b. group B alpha-hemolytic staphylococcus
   c. group C beta-hemolytic streptococcus
   d. group D alpha-hemolytic streptococcus

8. Older children are recommended to receive which vaccines? *(Select all that apply.)*
   a. DTaP
   b. Tdap
   c. PCV13
   d. HPV

9. Which vaccinations are given early in childhood?
   a. MMR
   b. Tdap
   c. HPV
   d. meningitis

10. _____ should not be given to children because of _____.
    a. Amoxicillin; sore throat
    b. Aspirin; Reye's syndrome
    c. Acetaminophen; acute otitis media
    d. Ibuprofen; fever

11. Which are ways to prevent administration errors in pediatric populations? *(Select all that apply.)*
    a. Have the caregiver use a teach-back.
    b. Use ordinary kitchen tablespoons for measuring.
    c. Counsel the caregiver with an administration demonstration.
    d. Use oral syringes with dosage markings.

12. When calculating a pediatric dose using Clark's Rule, we could take the adult dose:
    a. times the child's weight in pounds over 150.
    b. divided by the child's weight in pounds over 150.
    c. times 150 over the child's weight.
    d. times the child's weight in pounds over 50.

13. When using Young's Rule to calculate the dosage for a child, one would take the adult dose and:
    a. divide by 12.
    b. multiply by the age over the age + 12.
    c. multiply by 12.
    d. divide by the age over the age + 12.

14. Michael is 8 years old and weighs 75 lbs. He needs a dose of ibuprofen (7.5 mg/kg) for his fever. What is the dosage?
    a. 100 mg
    b. 128 mg
    c. 256 mg
    d. 300 mg

15. Aspirin given to children might cause which condition?
    a. Reye's syndrome
    b. arthritis
    c. inflammation
    d. fever

16. For an infant younger than 3 months, we would be concerned with a temperature at or above:
    a. 37° Celsius.
    b. 38° Celsius.
    c. 38.5° Celsius.
    d. 39° Celsius.

17. A child needs medication for fever; you would expect which two over-the-counter medications as options? *(Select all that apply.)*
    a. acetaminophen
    b. amoxicillin
    c. ibuprofen
    d. augmentin

18. The clavulanate in amoxicillin/clavulanate (Augmentin) serves as the:
    a. primary antibiotic.
    b. protection from bacterial enzymes.
    c. enzyme that degrades the bacteria.
    d. primary antiviral.

19. A patient with strep pharyngitis would first receive an antibiotic ending with _____ if they did not have a penicillin allergy.
    a. *-cillin*
    b. *-thromycin*
    c. *-methoxazole*
    d. *-mycin*

20. Common childhood vaccinations include all *except*:
    a. DTaP.
    b. rotavirus.
    c. PCV13.
    d. hepatitis C.

MATCHING TERMS (5)

Match the term to its definition or equivalent.

1. _____ middle ear infection
2. _____ age is used for dosing calculations
3. _____ weight is used for dosing calculations
4. _____ sore and inflamed throat
5. _____ when a majority of people are vaccinated

a. Clark's Rule
b. Young's Rule
c. acute otitis media
d. herd immunity
e. pharyngitis

MATCHING MEDICATIONS (5)

Match the item to the description.

1. _____ amoxicillin
2. _____ ibuprofen
3. _____ Clark's Rule
4. _____ Young's Rule
5. _____ DTaP

a. an age-based dosing calculation
b. a weight-based dosing calculation
c. pain reliever for fever and inflammation
d. antibiotic for infection
e. a type of vaccination

COMPLETION 1 (5)

1. _____ are considered less than 4 weeks old.

2. Weight-based dosing of _____ is 5-10 mg/kg/dose every 6-8 hours.

3. Weight-based dosing of _____ is 5-10 mg/kg/dose every 4-6 hours.

4. Due to Reye's syndrome, _____ can cause a severe reaction in children.

5. _____ younger than 3 months should be seen by a healthcare provider if they have a fever.

a. aspirin
b. neonates
c. ibuprofen
d. infants
e. acetaminophen

COMPLETION 2 (5)

1. A nonopioid analgesic that reduces fever. _____

2. An early childhood vaccination. _____

3. An antibiotic for non–penicillin-allergic patients. _____

4. An antibiotic for penicillin-allergic patients. _____

5. A severe reaction with aspirin in children. _____

a. Reye's syndrome
b. acetaminophen
c. amoxicillin
d. clindamycin
e. MMR

DOSAGE CALCULATIONS (10)

1. A 5-year-old child weighs 50 lbs. What dosage of ibuprofen does she need (7.5 mg/kg)?

2. Using Young's Rule, how many milligrams can a 6-year-old receive for an adult dose of 250 mg?

3. Using Clark's Rule, how many milligrams can a 30-lb child receive for an adult dose of 300 mg?

4. If a patient receives 5-10 mg/kg/dose of ibuprofen every 6 hours, what is the daily ibuprofen dose they can take?

5. If a patient who weighs 120 lbs needs to take acetaminophen 10-15 mg/kg/dose every 4 hours, what is the dosage range after 12 hours?

6. Using Clark's Rule, determine the pediatric dose with a 200-mg adult dose and a child who is 75 pounds.

7. Using Clark's Rule, determine the pediatric dose with a 100-mcg adult dose and a child who is 25 pounds.

8. Using Young's Rule, determine the pediatric dose with a 200-mg adult dose and a child who is 10 years old.

9. Using Young's Rule, determine the pediatric dose with a 100-mcg adult dose and a child who is 5 years old.

10. How many milligrams would a 22-pound patient receive if the dosage is 10 mg/kg/dose?

16 Geriatric Pharmacology

TRUE FALSE (10)

1. A person older than 65 years and another 30 years of age would experience similar health conditions. _____
2. The number of prescriptions decreases as a person gets older. _____
3. Once an adult reaches the 30-year-old mark, the cardiovascular system is affected. _____
4. There is no need for a dosage reduction when there is more drug in the body. _____
5. Aging can affect absorption, distribution, metabolism, and excretion. _____
6. A lipid-soluble drug has a longer half-life in the geriatric population. _____
7. Drugs act faster in the geriatric population because of increased blood flow to the GI tract. _____
8. Beers Criteria are used to assess the risk of medications used in older populations. _____
9. Metabolism increases as the person gets older. _____
10. The geriatric population has a slower drug excretion rate. _____

MULTIPLE CHOICE (10)

1. A person _____ or older is considered part of the geriatric population.
   a. 50
   b. 55
   c. 60
   d. 65

2. With increasing age, drug absorption is _____ because aging causes a(n) _____ drug action.
   a. faster; delayed
   b. slower; delayed
   c. faster; immediate
   d. slower; immediate

3. If an older patient takes _____ medications, _____ doses must be given because of changes in muscle mass and water.
   a. water-soluble; same
   b. fat-soluble; higher
   c. fat-soluble; lower
   d. water-soluble; higher

4. If a medication falls under the Beers Criteria, this indicates that it should be _____ for an older adult because of _____. *(Select all that apply.)*
   a. avoided; drug–drug interactions
   b. prescribed more; drug efficacy
   c. given immediately; time sensitivity
   d. used with caution; renal dose adjustments

5. The _____ affects with drug _____ and _____ significantly affect(s) drug _____.
   a. liver; metabolism; stomach; excretion
   b. stomach; metabolism; liver; excretion
   c. kidneys; metabolism; liver; excretion
   d. liver; metabolism; kidneys; excretion

6. A male patient's creatinine clearance is 60 mL. What would this value indicate and how would this affect dosing?
   a. It indicates the amount of creatinine that the body distributes per unit time, and there is a need to decrease the amount of drug given.
   b. It indicates the amount of creatinine that the liver metabolizes per unit time, and there is a need to increase the amount of drug given.
   c. It indicates the amount of creatinine that the kidneys excrete per unit time, and there is a need to decrease the amount of drug given.
   d. It indicates the amount of creatinine that the kidneys excrete per unit time, and there is a need to increase the amount of drug given.

7. How would you define physical dependence?
   a. The dose increases, yet the patient gets the same response.
   b. The dose decreases and the patient gets the same response.
   c. A condition of possible withdrawal after the abrupt discontinuation of a medication.
   d. The dose increases and the patient gets a heightened response.

8. What are some strategies to reduce the rate of noncompliance of medications in the geriatric population? *(Select all that apply.)*
   a. Increasing the prescribing cascade
   b. Deprescribing unnecessary medications
   c. Requesting non–child-proof caps
   d. Using a daily pill box

9. Which is true regarding the Beers Criteria?
   a. They are reviewed every 3 years by the American Geriatrics Society.
   b. They are reviewed every 5 years by the American Geriatrics Society.
   c. Changes in evidence do not lead to changes in the Beers Criteria.
   d. Changes in evidence do lead to changes in the Beers Criteria.

10. What is/are the common characteristic(s) in the geriatric population that can lead to poor distribution? *(Select all that apply.)*
    a. reduced kidney flow
    b. reduced total body water
    c. reduced plasma proteins
    d. reduced GI blood flow

MATCHING (5)

Match the related changes of the body to the geriatric population characteristics.

1. _____	absorption	a. increased in water retention
2. _____	excretion	b. reduced lean muscle mass
3. _____	distribution	c. reduced GI blood flow
4. _____	metabolism	d. reduced kidney blood flow
5. _____	hypertension	e. increased duration of drug action

COMPLETION (5)

1. For a patient diagnosed with benign prostatic hyperplasia, _____ can cause urinary retention.

2. Often, _____ can mask signs of hypoglycemia, which can be dangerous in those with diabetes.

3. In heart failure, if _____ is given, this can cause hypotension.

4. _____ given with diuretics can lead to cardiac arrhythmias.

5. A healthcare provider needs to reconsider recommending _____ for pain relief due to an increase in blood pressure.

a. propranolol
b. diphenhydramine
c. beta blockers
d. NSAIDs
e. digoxin

DOSAGE CALCULATIONS (5)

1. A patient is just diagnosed with hypertension and has acetaminophen, hydrochlorothiazide, propranolol, and furosemide on their chart. Which medication should be deprescribed?

2. In the patient's medication chart, propranolol, verapamil, diltiazem, metoprolol, and ibuprofen are listed. Which medications represent therapeutic duplications?

3. Which of these changes affect the geriatric population: increased GI blood flow, low lean muscle mass, decreased metabolism, and increased kidney blood flow?

4. Which of these characteristics are used to prevent medication toxicity in the geriatric population using the Beers Criteria: age, disease states, renal function, polypharmacy, and compliance?

5. Which of these drug classes should be taken into consideration with other comorbidities in the geriatric population: first-generation beta blockers, NSAIDs, diuretics, and anticholinergics?

VISUAL CRITICAL THINKING (1)

1. How can this device help geriatric patients? What is another possible way to improve compliance?

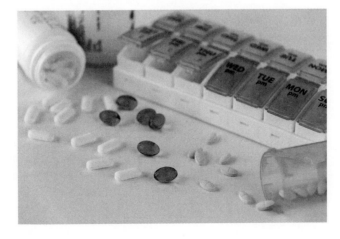

17 Local and General Anesthetics

TRUE FALSE (10)

1. Local anesthetics activate fast voltage-gated potassium channels of sensory neurons. _____
2. Etidocaine is one example of a local amide anesthetic. _____
3. An acidic environment allows molecules to be more unionized, which will enable local anesthetics to cross the barrier. _____
4. When the partition coefficient is lower, the drug is more potent. _____
5. One possible organ affected by anesthetic effects is the heart. _____
6. Memories are not triggered when using general anesthetics. _____
7. Stage four of anesthesia is when unconsciousness and regular breathing occur. _____
8. When anesthetics are given intravenously, there is fast recovery. _____
9. Non-barbiturates such as dexmedetomidine can be used to induce anesthesia. _____
10. CNS effects are rare with the use of general anesthesia. _____

MULTIPLE CHOICE (10)

1. Which are ester local anesthetics? *(Select all that apply.)*
   a. lidocaine
   b. procaine
   c. tetracaine
   d. chloroprocaine

2. A patient has an allergy to procaine. Which should the prescriber use instead? *(Select all that apply.)*
   a. lidocaine
   b. bupivacaine
   c. tetracaine
   d. chloroprocaine

3. In a(n) _____ environment, the molecules will be more _____, and it will _____.
   a. acidic; unionized; not cross the barrier
   b. basic; ionized; cross the barrier
   c. basic; unionized; cross the barrier
   d. acidic; unionized; not cross the barrier

4. When an anesthetic has a high partition coefficient, there is _____ and _____.
   a. high lipophilicity; long half-life
   b. high lipophilicity; short half-life
   c. low lipophilicity; long half-life
   d. low lipophilicity; short half-life

5. Common adverse effects of anesthetics are: *(Select all that apply.)*
   a. arrhythmias.
   b. metallic taste.
   c. delirium.
   d. euphoria.

6. The body excretes _____ local anesthetics unchanged through the kidney, but _____ local anesthetics are broken down, resulting in PABA production.
   a. ester; acetyl
   b. amide; ester
   c. ester; amide
   d. acetyl; ester

7. With pregnant patients, the preferred local anesthetic prescribers should use is:
   a. chloroprocaine.
   b. etidocaine.
   c. prilocaine.
   d. lidocaine.

8. Which stage of anesthesia involves medullary depression?
   a. stage one
   b. stage two
   c. stage three
   d. stage four

9. Which drug classes can be used as adjunct medications? *(Select all that apply.)*
   a. anticholinergics
   b. antibacterials
   c. antianxiety
   d. anticonvulsants

10. In addition to the use of local anesthetics, a _____ is added to increase the duration of action, allowing the drug to stay longer in the body before clearance.
    a. vasodilator
    b. vasoconstrictor
    c. bronchodilator
    d. bronchoconstrictor

MATCHING (5)

Match the description to the stage of anesthesia or property of the local anesthetic.

1. _____ delirium
2. _____ analgesia
3. _____ decreased eye movement
4. _____ longer half-life
5. _____ medullary depression

a. stage one
b. stage two
c. stage three
d. stage four
e. high partition coefficient

COMPLETION (5)

1. A(n) _____ may be used for procedures by itself that do not require a long duration.

2. The use of _____ depends on the concentration gradient from the lung alveoli to the blood and into the brain.

3. Because _____ have a lower partition coefficient, they are less potent.

4. Often, as a general anesthetic, _____ provide sedation and its other component reduces flammability.

5. _____ are not used often due to more allergic reactions to the PABA metabolite.

a. amide local anesthetics
b. ester local anesthetics
c. inhaled oral anesthetic
d. intravenous anesthetic
e. halogenated hydrocarbons

96

Chapter **17** **Local and General Anesthetics**

DOSAGE CALCULATIONS (5)

1. From this local anesthetics list: lidocaine, procaine, tetracaine, bupivacaine, and etidocaine, which are amide local anesthetics?

2. From this list of effects: disorientation, ringing in ears, amnesia, seizures, and delirium, which are signs of the stages of anesthetics and not a side effect?

3. Based on these classes of medications: antiarrhythmics, anticholinergics, antiallergy, and antianxiety, which are used as adjunct medications to treat adverse effects?

4. If a local anesthetic drug A partition coefficient is 5 and a local anesthetic drug B partition coefficient is 2, which one should the prescriber use for a shorter duration of action?

5. Tetracaine takes about 8 hours to take effect. Since tetracaine takes about four times longer than procaine, how much time does it take for procaine to take effect?

VISUAL CRITICAL THINKING (6)

1. Mechanisms of opioid action in the spinal cord. Place the terms *blocked, calcium, cAMP, neuron, nociceptors,* and *potassium* in the figure.

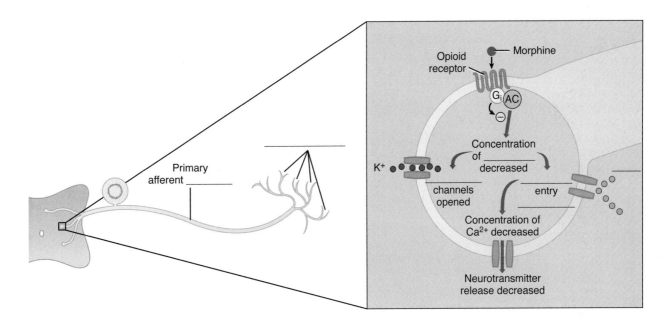

2. How Local Anesthetics Work. Place the terms *active, amino, carboxy, inactive,* and *resting* in the figure.

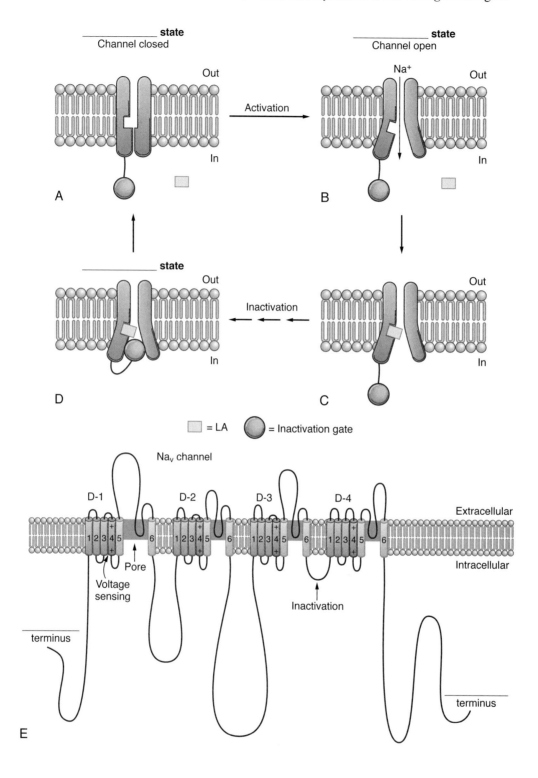

3. Amides versus Esters. Place the terms *lidocaine* and *procaine* in the figure.

	Structure	pKa	Ionization at pH 7.4 (%)	Partition coefficient	Protein bound (%)
Ester type					
_____	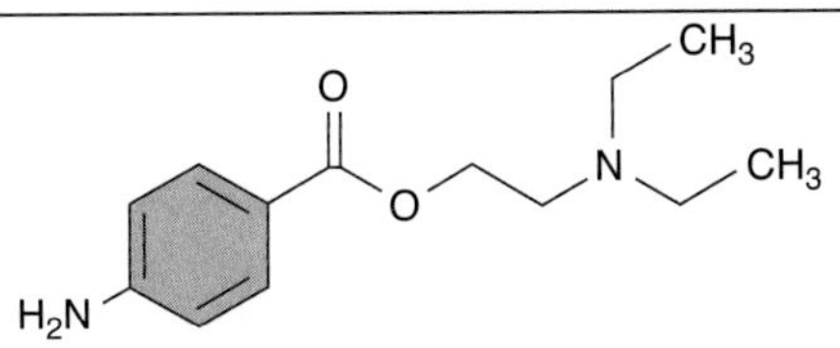	8.9	97	100	6
Tetracaine	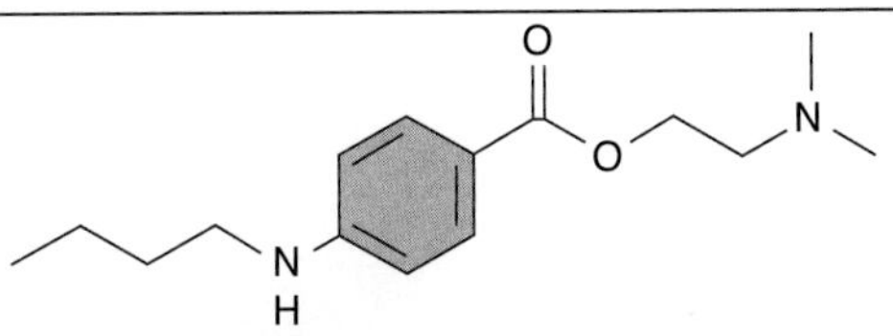	8.5	93	5822	76
Chloroprocaine	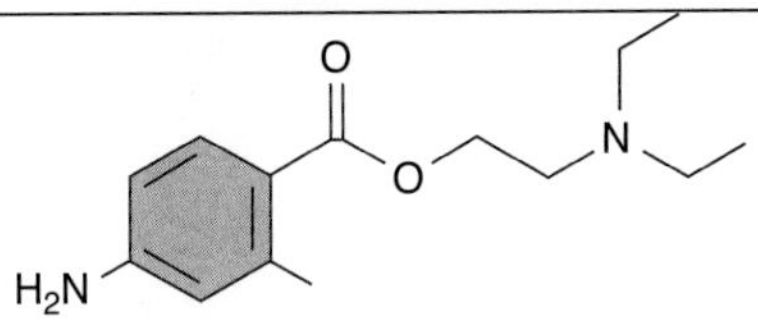	9.1	95	810	N/A
Amide type					
_____	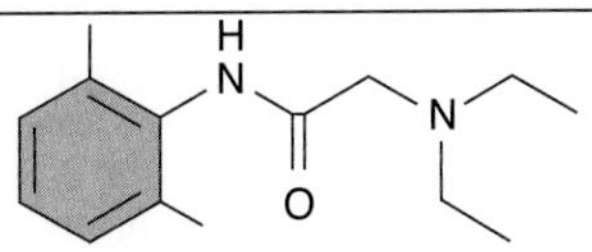	7.9	76	366	65
Prilocaine	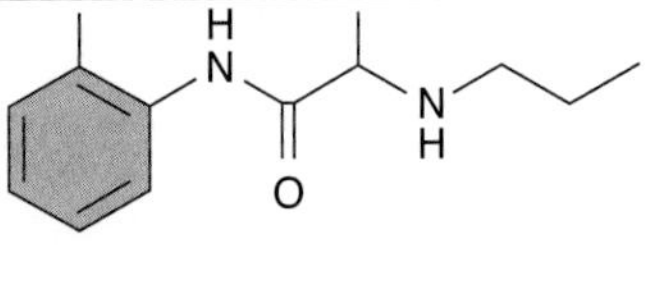	7.9	76	129	55
Ropivacaine	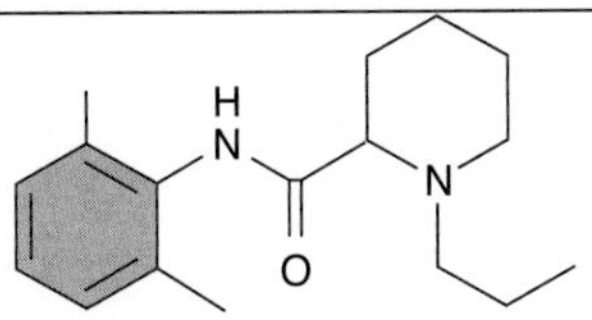	8.1	83	775	94

4. Epidural Administration. Place the terms *body, ganglion,* and *process* in the figure.

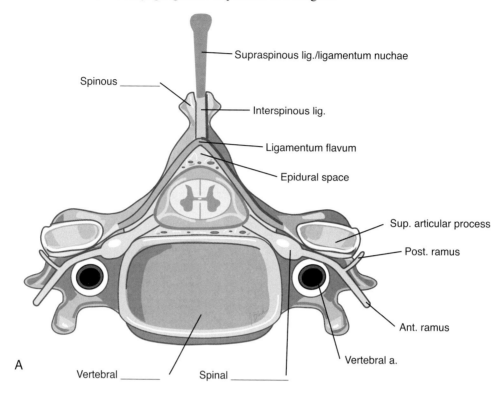

Supraspinous lig./ligamentum nuchae

Spinous _____

Interspinous lig.

Ligamentum flavum

Epidural space

Sup. articular process

Post. ramus

Ant. ramus

Vertebral a.

A

Vertebral _____   Spinal _____

5. Midsagittal Section through the Spinal Column. Place the terms *body, equina,* and *space* in the figure.

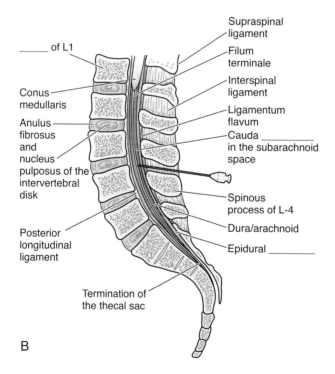

_____ of L1

Conus medullaris

Anulus fibrosus and nucleus pulposus of the intervertebral disk

Posterior longitudinal ligament

Termination of the thecal sac

Supraspinal ligament

Filum terminale

Interspinal ligament

Ligamentum flavum

Cauda _____ in the subarachnoid space

Spinous process of L-4

Dura/arachnoid

Epidural _____

B

6. Horizontal Section through the Body of L3. Place the terms *body, dura,* and *epidural* in the figure.

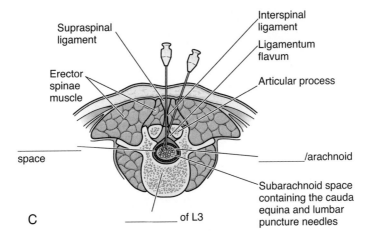

Supraspinal ligament

Erector spinae muscle

Interspinal ligament

Ligamentum flavum

Articular process

_____ space

_____/arachnoid

Subarachnoid space containing the cauda equina and lumbar puncture needles

C

_____ of L3

18 Alcohol and Drugs of Abuse

TRUE FALSE (10)

1. Substance use disorder is only the abuse of illegal substances. _____
2. Withdrawal symptoms occur when one stops chronic alcohol or tobacco use. _____
3. One method of treatment in smoking cessation includes behavioral therapy. _____
4. Opioids release serotonin throughout the body and may cause addiction. _____
5. Drugs like diazepam and triazolam do not have the potential for abuse. _____
6. There is a significant increase in dopamine after the use of methamphetamines. _____
7. There is no treatment available for those at risk of an overdose of opioids. _____
8. Alcohol use disorder can lead to liver disease, digestion problems, and heart disease. _____
9. Campral can be used to keep a patient from drinking by making alcohol less rewarding. _____
10. The withdrawal symptoms are what make dependence challenging to overcome. _____

MULTIPLE CHOICE (10)

1. Which best describes how drugs of abuse affect dependence?
   a. Dependence occurs because drugs of abuse operate in an adrenaline pathway to create a feeling of elation.
   b. Dependence does not occur because there are no withdrawal symptoms from drugs of abuse.
   c. Dependence does not occur because drugs of abuse can be used as a treatment.
   d. Dependence occurs because drugs of abuse operate in the reward pathway to create a feeling of elation.

2. How long after the cessation of chronic alcohol consumption would one expect to see signs of hallucinations?
   a. 6 hours
   b. 12 hours
   c. 24 hours
   d. 48 hours

3. A patient is taking medication for chronic alcohol disorder. Each time they drink alcohol, they now get a nauseating reaction that deters them from drinking alcohol again. What medication is this patient taking?
   a. disulfiram
   b. acamprosate
   c. naltrexone
   d. bupropion

4. In what way can naltrexone be used in chronic alcoholic disorder?
   a. as medically supervised detoxification
   b. as a euphoria blocker in alcohol use disorder
   c. as an overdose reversal if given right away
   d. to reduce cravings for alcohol

5. What options are available for those who want to quit smoking? *(Select all that apply.)*
   a. buprenorphine
   b. bupropion
   c. nicotine patch
   d. nicotine lozenge

6. A patient indicates nicotine replacement therapy (NRT) did not work for them and asks for prescription recommendations. Which can be recommended to help them with smoking cessation?
   a. eszopiclone
   b. varenicline
   c. buprenorphine
   d. morphine

7. Naloxone can be used to treat overdose for which drug(s)? *(Select all that apply.)*
   a. nicotine
   b. heroin
   c. bupropion
   d. fentanyl

8. In chronic opioid use, what can occur? *(Select all that apply.)*
   a. fast breathing
   b. slow breathing
   c. constipation
   d. diarrhea

9. Opioid withdrawal commonly involves: *(Select all that apply.)*
   a. hot flashes.
   b. cold flashes.
   c. diarrhea.
   d. bone pain.

10. Medications such as lorazepam and alprazolam can have high abuse potential. If a patient undergoes an overdose of these types of medications, which should the patient be given?
    a. naltrexone
    b. naloxone
    c. buprenorphine
    d. flumazenil

MATCHING (5)

Match the medication to the indication.

1.	_____	naltrexone
2.	_____	acamprosate
3.	_____	disulfiram
4.	_____	bupropion
5.	_____	buprenorphine

a. keeps one from drinking by reacting with any alcohol, causing an unpleasant reaction
b. for decreasing severity of cravings
c. for alcohol use disorder to block euphoria of alcohol
d. for heroin withdrawal
e. for smoking cessation aid

COMPLETION (5)

1. _____ causes the development of various diseases such as heart disease, liver disease, and problems with vision and sexual function.
2. While _____ can be used for smoking cessation, it cannot be used in seizure disorders.
3. _____ comes in the form of patches, gum, and lozenges to aid in smoking cessation.
4. To reverse an opioid overdose, _____ can be given either as an intranasal spray or an intramuscular injection.
5. Hand tremors, seizures, and high blood pressure are among the _____ once stopping chronic alcohol use.

a. withdrawal symptoms
b. alcohol use disorder
c. bupropion
d. nicotine replacement therapy
e. Narcan

DOSAGE CALCULATIONS (5)

1. Among these drugs: oxycodone, hydrocodone, codeine, and buprenorphine, which would lead to a possible overdose, and can Narcan be used to reverse the overdose?

2. A patient comes in with shaking hands, anxiety, and headache, but soon the patient becomes more disoriented, then they start having seizures. How many hours has it been based on the general progression of withdrawal symptoms?

3. Which of these drugs: Campral, Antabuse, Narcan, Zyban, and Chantix, are used to treat various withdrawal symptoms of alcohol disorder?

4. Out of these drugs: naloxone, bupropion, buprenorphine, methadone, codeine, lorazepam used for withdrawal and treatment of substance abuse disorder, which are typically used for heroin withdrawal?

5. Which of these drugs: alprazolam, diazepam, triazolam, naloxone, and marijuana, are considered benzodiazepines with high potential for abuse?

VISUAL CRITICAL THINKING (2)

1. Overdose Death Rates Involving Opioids. Place the terms *any, commonly,* and *heroin* in the figure.

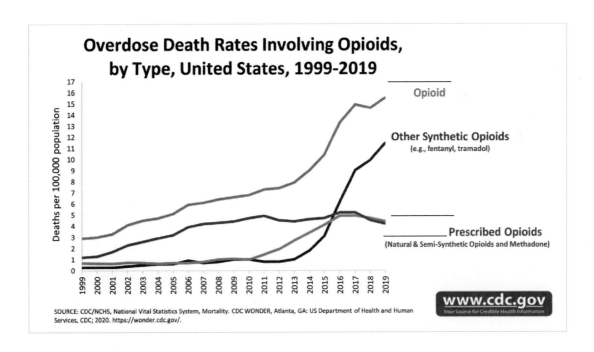

2. Commonly Prescribed Benzodiazapines. Place the terms *Alprazolam, Ativan, Chlordiazepoxide, Clonazepam, Halcion, Restoril,* and *Valium* in the figure.

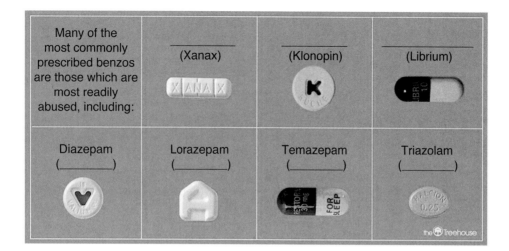

Many of the most commonly prescribed benzos are those which are most readily abused, including:	(Xanax)	(Klonopin)	(Librium)
Diazepam (_____)	Lorazepam (_____)	Temazepam (_____)	Triazolam (_____)

Notes

Notes